Also by Marla Cilley
*Sink Reflections*

Also by Leanne Ely
*Saving Dinner*

# Body Clutter

*love your body, love yourself*

Marla Cilley—The FlyLady

Leanne Ely—The Dinner Diva

A Fireside Book
Published by Simon & Schuster
New York   London   Toronto   Sydney

This publication contains the opinions and ideas of its authors. It is intended to provide helpful and informative material on the subjects addressed in the publication. It is sold with the understanding that the authors and publisher are not engaged in rendering medical, health, or any other kind of personal professional services in the book. The reader should consult his or her medical, health, or other competent professional before adopting any of the suggestions in this book or drawing inferences from it.

The authors and publisher specifically disclaim all responsibility for any liability, loss or risk, personal or otherwise, which is incurred as a consequence, directly or indirectly, of the use and application of any of the contents of this book.

FIRESIDE
Rockefeller Center
1230 Avenue of the Americas
New York, New York 10020

First Fireside Edition September 2006

FIRESIDE and colophon are registered trademarks
of Simon & Schuster, Inc.

For information regarding special discounts for bulk purchases,
please contact Simon & Schuster Special Sales at
1-800-456-6798 or business@simonandschuster.com.

Designed and typeset by Naomi Rosenblatt and Shey Wolvek-Pfister of
HelioTrope Graphics, New York City

Cover design concept by Stephanie Burns

Edited by Kelly Burns

Manufactured in the United States of America

10   9   8   7   6   5

Library of Congress Cataloging-in-Publication Data
Cilley, Marla
    Body clutter : love your body, love yourself / Marla Cilley, Leanne Ely.—
    1st Fireside ed.
        p. cm
    Originally published: Brevard, N.C. : Flylady & Co., © 2005
    1. Appetite disorders. 2. Food—Psychological aspects. 3. Weight loss.
    4. Nutrition. 5. Health. I. Ely, Leanne. II. Title.

    RC552.E18C495 2006b
    613.2—dc22

                                                            2006050138

ISBN-13: 978-1-4165-3462-4
ISBN-10:       1-4165-3462-8

*This book is lovingly dedicated to all of the FlyBabies and Menu-Mailerettes who have suffered in silence, thinking they were the only ones who have struggled and desperately wanted to release their Body Clutter.*

# Contents

# CONTENTS

# Acknowledgments

Dear Friends,

No book is complete till we thank the people who helped give birth to our labor of love. The idea of Body Clutter was conceived during a month when we were focusing on moving and nutrition on the FlyLady website. We had written several essays dealing with food, nutrition, exercise, and getting rid of our stinking thinking. We decided that we might actually have a book that our members desperately needed. We instant-messaged each other with our ideas; we talked for hours on the phone and created an outline. And before we knew it, the book started to take shape.

We are SHEs. We get so easily bored with the process. We are filled with inspiration, but then, when the enthusiasm subsides, we are left with an unfinished project. In order to breathe some life back into our words, we begged Kelly to take on the daunting task of taking our words and turning them into a book. That was the real birthing process.

We had gone through the excitement of wanting to do a book, just like a woman does when she decides that she wants to have a baby. We had the idea, an outline, several chapters, but we didn't know what to do next. We needed a birthing coach. Kelly was the one person who pushed us when we needed pushing. She pulled things out of us when we were not willing to release our own Body Clutter, and she gave us hope that one day we would have a book to present to the world.

Every member of the FLY crew and Saving Dinner crew has cheered us on and helped us by taking on some of our chores so we would have more time to devote to our labor of love, *Body Clutter*. Robert, Tom, Justin, Jack, Michele, Rebecca, Wendy, Misty, Carolyn S., Paddi, Jessica, Kathy, Laura, Lee, Dana, Chris H., Katie, Jim, Michael, Darlena, Naomi, Shey, Alice, Sandy, Carolyn P., Emily, Ethan, Stephanie, T.J., Alexander, Courtney, Christopher P., Caroline, Peter, Miriam, Bonnie, Robyn, and Kandi—we give to all of you our heartfelt gratitude and thanks. To our FlyBabies and Menu-Mailerettes around the world, we thank you for asking us for this book, patiently waiting for it to come to life, for supporting us, and for being the reason that we do what we do.

This book had a life of its own. It was going to be born one way or another. The last months were tough, as with any birthing process. We could actually visualize our due date, but did we really have to go through the process every single day to get there? What else did we have to do; couldn't this be easier? Kelly told us that the reason we were struggling so with the book is that we were living a lie. We were not walking the walk. We could talk the talk, but we had to come face-to-face with our own Body Clutter if this book was going to come to life. Did we mention that she is one tough editor?

Even that was not enough for us. It took major personal health emergencies to get our attention. The fact was we were two people struggling with our own Body Clutter. What example could we be to the world if we were not taking care of ourselves? The book took on a newfound motivation; we began to take the BabySteps we were teaching and apply them to our lives. We started to see results.

Here we are with a finished book, but the book is not what was really born. It was through the journey that we took, not in the writing of the book but in taking our own words and applying them to our lives, that the book *Body Clutter* has actually given birth to us. You can take this journey, too, one BabyStep at a time. Read each page and start your own journey through the birthing process to discover the YOU who is hiding behind your Body Clutter.

We love you all,
*FlyLady* and *Leanne*

# Foreword

Dear Friends,

I was given the ultimate honor of helping FlyLady and Leanne give birth to their labor of love, *Body Clutter*. What a labor it has been! When they asked me to join in on this life-changing event I was not prepared for the journey that I was about to embark on. I read what they had written so far and, while I liked the content, I did not love the book. There was so much more that these amazing women had to share, but they were not quite prepared to share it. When I first started working with them and asked questions, they would give me some very nice pat answers, but I wanted more because I knew that you would ask for more.

I relate this to the questions I get asked about the missions that I write for the FlyLady mentoring list. I am always asked, "Just how do you know that I need to (fill in the blank)?" The reason I know is that they are things that I need to do myself. Just as when I started asking FlyLady and Leanne questions, it was because I knew that you the reader would ask the same things. As time went by and the phone calls were getting longer and longer, I came to an astounding realization: FlyLady and Leanne are powerful women, helping thousands around the globe change their homes and lives, but they were underestimating their power to change their own lives.

As I continued to badger them, hunt them down on cell phones, and basically pound them over the head with my questions and arguments of why they had to answer me, we started to really bring this book into shape. As I dug deeper and deeper into their minds and hearts, they began to question themselves. We ended up having phone calls that were truly therapy sessions. We would talk about all the diet books, plans, etc., on the market and how they don't work. I remember interrupting a tirade on these books and saying very simply, "Actually, they all work as long as you do them." Just so you know, it is not often that FlyLady and Leanne are silent. What I said that day rendered them speechless . . . but only for a moment! That was a lightbulb moment and the beginning of a turning point for all of us. This book had to show you how to really dig deep within yourselves to find out how you found the weight, not just how to lose it.

That is when we started working on uncharted territory for FlyLady and Leanne. This book was not just about BabySteps and how to apply the FlyLady system to your Body Clutter. There were deep-rooted emotional issues that had to be addressed as well. I started giving them assignments so they could BabyStep through this process—and we were on a roll! We thought we were on our way, but then we all started to get burned out and needed to take a break. During that time, I was still paying close attention to FlyLady and Leanne—how they talked, what they said, what they wrote—and I came to a big conclusion: It wasn't that we were burned out, it was that they were not living what they were writing about, or to use their words, they were talking the talk, but not walking the walk. There was a tear-filled conversation and the beginning of a new chapter, not just in this book but also in our lives.

There were moments of laughter, tears, arguments, and a few yelling matches, but our goal was always to share with you this amazing process of releasing your Body Clutter, not just from your backside and thighs but from between your ears as well. We went through some health scares along the way that you will read about in the book and had to peel back the layers of defense shields that had been in place for so long. We have come to the end of our writing journey and are now ready to invite you along for the ride.

As you begin your journey into Body Clutter, please know that every single word, sentence, paragraph, and chapter has been created expressly for those of you who have been suffering and living in silent torment over your Body Clutter. I promise that when you have finished this book you will have been on an amazing ride that will take you on to your own personal journey—to FLY!

*Kelly*

# *Glossary*

## *of Special Words and Terms Used Throughout This Book*

**BabySteps**. BabySteps are small steps so you take your time instead of getting burned out and wanting too much too fast. We have to learn how to take small BabySteps and put them together to make up some routines.

**Before Bed Routine**. The most important routine of the whole day. Getting prepared the night before starts you in the right direction for the next morning.

**Bless Your Heart**. This is what we lovingly call exercise. When we move, we are blessing our hearts.

**BO**. Born Organized.

**CHAOS.** *Can't Have Anyone Over Syndrome*. The fear of allowing anyone into your home because of the chaos that has taken over.

**Control Journal.** A FlyLady tool that is customized by you to help you stay on track with your daily routines and activities.

**DD.** Dear Daughter.

**DH.** Dear Husband.

**DS.** Dear Son.

**Five-Minute Room Rescue.** A tool that is used in the FlyLady system to help you tackle a small area in the most chaotic room in your home. You rescue this room five minutes at a time.

**FLY & FLYing.** Finally Loving Yourself.

**FlyBabies.** New members to the FlyLady system are called FlyBabies. As a FlyBaby, you are just getting started. You are never behind and can jump in where you are.

**Franny.** A symbol of the sad person within us all when we are surrounded by CHAOS.

**free radicals.** Kind of like body pollution. Your body produces free radicals when you breathe. They can damage cells and age you prematurely unless you have enough antioxidants to combat them. Antioxidants: like the Pac-Men of free radicals. Antioxidants are nutrients (like vitamins A and E) that scavange for free radicals in the body.

**God Breeze**. Imagine God as being the picture of that ole north wind. Then he puffs out His cheeks to blow a breeze in your direction. Then imagine that you are sitting in a tiny sailboat on a still lake and the breeze comes in your direction. You can put your sails up and allow the breeze to send you in its direction, or you can do nothing and sit dead in the water.

**HALT**. Don't allow yourself to get too Hungry, Angry, Lonely, or Tired.

**Hot Spot**. Any area in your home that as soon as it is clean becomes covered up again with clutter.

**Morning Routine**. This is the compilation of small BabySteps that you take to establish as a habit when you first get up in the morning.

**phytochemicals**. Teeny tiny plant chemicals (found in fruit and vegetables) that lower your risk of cancer.

**SHE**™. This is a concept from *Sidetracked Home Executives: From Pigpen to Paradise* by Pam Young and Peggy Jones. They came up with the underlying principles of the FlyLady system and have endorsed the way it is taught.

**Sidetracked**. We start one thing and go to another, then do not finish what we started in the first place.

**Stinking Thinking**. The negative thoughts going round and round in our head.

**27-Fling Boogie**. A tool used in the FlyLady system to help declutter your home.

# Introduction

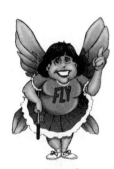

FlyLady

What is Body Clutter, anyway? When you look at your house, sometimes you can see the clutter. Then there are times when you are immune to your clutter; it can be right in front of you and you don't see it. It starts gradually slipping in your door while the other stuff you already have is just waiting to be loved. Eventually clutter gains a foothold and you don't know where to start to get rid of it. It seems like such an overwhelming task; what is a person supposed to do with all this stuff?

Over the years, the same thing has happened to our body. As children, our little child brain and body absorbed every word and morsel of food that came even close to us. We were starving for knowledge and attention, and our tiny body needed love, food, and movement to continue to grow. Some of the messages told us that we could have it "all," while others said, "If you don't do it right, don't do it at all." We were stuck wanting it "all" and afraid even to try because what if we failed? Then you toss in the time factor of perfectionism and you will find the ultimate killer of souls: procrastination. "I don't have time!" That is, we don't have time to do it right, so we do nothing at all.

This thought process is part of our Body Clutter. It is one of our many attitudes that have helped us to collect the clutter that is on our thighs, tummy, and backside. Just like with our homes, our body did not become cluttered overnight. It took years of stinking thinking to collect our Body Clutter. It happened so gradually that the only time we really noticed was when we had to reach for a larger dress size. Do you remember the horror the first time you got a bigger size? Are you immune to it now?

This book is not one of those magic pills you have been searching for. It has been a difficult journey for us, but we have celebrated every BabyStep we have taken. With each step we have released some of our negative thinking and with it the hold on our physical Body Clutter.

Over the years we have collectively lost and gained millions of pounds; we are good at starving ourselves and losing the weight when we are forced into decluttering for a special occasion. Anytime you declutter for the wrong reasons, the clutter is going to come back and usually increase. We have all done the stash-and-dash around the house to get ready for a visit from our mother-in-law. That is what we do to our body, too.

The age-old problem for anyone who has ever been on a

"diet" is how to keep the pounds off once you are no longer depriving yourself. Leanne and I believe with all our hearts that the answer to this problem is not in the future but in the past. If we can figure out for ourselves how we acquired the Body Clutter in the first place and the attitude that put it there, then we are a step closer to eliminating it from our body. If we declutter the negative thinking first, it is going to help us stop gaining more Body Clutter. Then, by replacing our negative thought patterns with positive ones, we will gradually decrease the Body Clutter we already have.

Here is what happens when we don't declutter our negative attitudes. We decide to lose weight for whatever reason, we lose a few pounds, then something upsets us and we fall back into our old childhood habits of reaching for a "comfort cookie." It happened to me just the other day. I got my feelings hurt and I cried. I was crushed, and the first thought I had was to look in the freezer for a chocolate ice pop. What made me do that? It was almost instinctive! Immediately I saw it for what it was: a Band-Aid to comfort my hurting soul. This is how I used to deal with my hurt feelings; I would head to the refrigerator to stuff my face so I would not have to deal with what was really wrong. Before, I would not have been able to stop myself because I didn't know that my eating in response to feeling hurt was just as abusive as the comment that hurt my feelings in the first place. I just wanted to feel better and stop crying. This kind of behavior is not only instinctive but also very human.

When we are babies and we cry, what happens? We get

fed. When we misbehave in the grocery store, we are given a cookie to keep us quiet. Do you see the pattern here? It starts out as instinctual but ends up creating a pattern for self-destructive behavior. We are going to learn to recognize this Body Clutter for what it is—self-abuse.

Several years ago I began to FLY (Finally Loving Yourself), but it did not happen overnight. In fact, I am still learning how to love myself in almost every area of my life. My first BabySteps were about getting rid of the clutter and CHAOS (Can't Have Anyone Over Syndrome) in my life. I wanted to feel good about my home, but that is really hard to do when you are not feeling good about yourself.

It all started with shining my sink, and from that starting point, I began to take better care of my outward appearance, too. There is just something about walking into the bathroom and smiling at what you see in the mirror. It is kind of like going into your kitchen the morning after you have shined your sink for the first time—that smile radiates to the core of your being and it continues to surprise you each time you go into the kitchen and see your shining sink. Body Clutter is painful. Leanne and I have both suffered from the ridicule and snide comments. Those hurtful words and looks do not make us who we are. We wrote this book to help you find peace. Peace with food, movement, and, most of all, the attitude that has created your Body Clutter. We look in your faces and know that you are suffering just like we are. This book is our journey. It is because of you that we were able to address our own Body Clutter, and we thank you for that. We have given you our hearts and pray that our journey will help you release your own Body Clutter.

Leanne

I have struggled with my weight since the birth of my first child. The battle began after I gained more than fifty pounds with my daughter, and then gave birth to my son less than two years later. At that point my weight became more of a concern than I ever wanted it to be.

I had lost a baby the prior year to miscarriage, so when I found out I was pregnant with my daughter, I was determined to be the healthiest pregnant mom on the planet. First up on my be-healthy list was my diet. Prepregnancy, I ate erratically and only when my blood sugar crashed, and when I did eat I would pig out. I was a very picky eater who didn't like vegetables, but I trained myself to eat all of them —and like them! I ate regular meals but was overcome by the myth of eating for two and continued to pig out at each meal as if it were my last. Sundays after church became an excuse to belly up to a double cheeseburger, sides of fries and onion rings, and don't forget the chocolate shake! That was my splurge day, never mind that I had been splurging all week! I gained fifty-two pounds and ultimately gave birth to a nearly ten-pound baby.

With my second pregnancy, a new interest in nutrition helped keep my weight gain down to a manageable twenty-seven pounds. Unfortunately, the previous pregnancy's weight was still firmly in place.

I decided to become a nutritionist right after the birth of my son. The funny thing is that at the time I wasn't even interested in nutrition for myself. I just wanted to raise my children in a healthy manner.

The certification course I was taking would normally take two years to complete, but it took me only six months. My mentors, whom the school assigns its students, couldn't believe I was going through everything so rapidly, but I was determined to get it done ASAP so I would be qualified to feed my children healthy meals, as well as help other mothers with nutrition issues.

In between taking care of two babies, I studied twelve hours a day, often staying up till one or two in the morning. It was awful, but I did get my certification, I did feed my children an unbelievably healthy diet, and I began taking clients for consultations, and speaking to preschools and anyone who would book me. I was on a crusade to tell the world how to feed their children, and yet my bottom continued to bloom into plus sizes. Ironically, I knew that I was talking the talk and not walking the walk, yet at the time it was all about the children.

The interesting thing about Body Clutter is that it's always there for a reason. It isn't just about overeating or not getting enough exercise. The reasons can vary, but getting to the heart of the matter and finding out why the Body Clutter is there in the first place can be the first step toward liberation. FlyLady and I, and more and more women just like us, are finding this out for ourselves; we have embarked on a journey together and the lightbulbs of enlightenment are going on all over the place. We want to share with you what we have discovered and have been implementing along the way.

One of the most comforting things I learned was that who I am does not equal my dress size. I am a unique woman, a child of God, with talents, gifts, and abilities that reach beyond the superficiality of size. I hope that when I'm gone, the things said about me will never be about my weight, the size of my jeans, or what color lipstick I wore. Instead, I hope they will say things about my character and that I was a good mom and a good friend. I am blessed with friends and family who love me as I am.

However, there is always room for improvement. One of the neatest things about the journey of life is the ability to redefine oneself. Self-assessment can be painful at times, but all growing pains lead to growth, which is the important thing. If we are not growing, we are stagnating and, to me, that's a fate worse than death.

So we go forward on the journey, recognizing that it is a learning process, an opportunity for growth, and that it may be painful at times. Sometimes the progress is amazing and noticeable; other times, it's one step forward and ten steps back. With the right tools, attitude, and a little knowledge, we can go all the way and really learn how to FLY— without the baggage!

## Body Clutter Mission

To help release your Body Clutter, we want you to use this book as a tool and take the words to heart. While you are reading you will need to have a few items right beside you. Keep in mind that this is your book and you can write in it and highlight all you want.

So right now go grab a pen, a highlighter, and a notebook. It doesn't matter what kind of notebook you find as long it has empty pages in it. Don't allow your perfectionism to keep you from using what you have around the house. This is your Body Clutter Control Journal. You will see with each Mission how quickly it will become your best friend.

Your Body Clutter journey starts now.

# 1. Food: The Ultimate Weapon of Self-Destruction

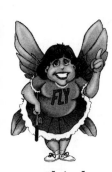

*FlyLady*

None of us can deny that at times we have used food as a drug. It may not be our drug of choice, but it is always handy: that drive-thru window, your microwave, the refrigerator or pantry. Food has been there for us from the time we were in our mother's arms to the present. We cried and we got a bottle, the breast, or a cookie put in front of us. It is kind of like training a puppy—it is usually done with a treat. We are no different, and guess what? It is not our fault.

Food is our comfort zone—when we have a full tummy, we feel content. Just like when we were babies, we would stop crying when our tummy was full and satisfied. Several years ago I used to stuff my face to keep from crying my eyes out. The more I stuffed food down my throat, the more I was pushing away dealing with the real prob-

1

lems. I still have to face the results of that overdose on food each time I see myself in the mirror. After many years of loving me just the way I am, I have finally realized that it was the emotional pain that I had never dealt with that put the Body Clutter on me.

Even after getting rid of the problems, my size did not change. It is much easier to put the Body Clutter on than it is to eliminate it, so much so that I finally gave up on the d-word (diet) and accepted me exactly as I am. That stopped the self-punishment of the crash-and-burn diets and my yo-yo weight. My weight has been stable now for a very long time.

I can still use food as a drug. I may not be stuffing my bad feelings like I used to, but it is still a habit that is very hard to break. Even happy moments are celebrated over a plate of food; we all do this and it is not wrong. The first step, and the hardest part, is realizing why we are eating and how much we are eating.

We all have foods that trigger some kind of past experience in us. Think about it right now: What food do you absolutely love so much that you cannot get enough of it? For me it is macaroni and cheese. If I have any left over in the refrigerator, it won't be there long; I can't wait to get back to the bowl. It doesn't matter if it is cold or hot, I want to eat it until it is all gone. I cannot ever remember getting my fill, even when I ate the whole thing. So, I ask myself, "What is going on here?"

I started looking at why I could not be satisfied with

normal and healthy portions of certain foods, and kept digging into my childhood. I finally got my answer. I remembered that during the summer between the fifth and sixth grades I stayed with my mother while my sisters visited our father. It was also the summer that I went to three different camps. Between sessions, I came home to an absentee parent and not much food in the house. All I could scavenge was a bag of elbow macaroni and a can of cream of cheddar soup. I was old enough to know a little about cooking, so I cooked the whole bag of macaroni and put the can of cheese soup in it. It was all I had—the food was my only friend.

The bowl of mac and cheese filled my feelings of rejection, abandonment, and loneliness. If I could not feel full of love and peace, I could at least feel full and that comforted me temporarily. I still hurt thinking about that time. I know in my heart that everything that has ever happened to me has made me who I am today. But at least I am not reaching for that bowl as I let myself experience that pain right now.

Have you figured out what that certain food is for you? It could be ice cream, potato chips, or chocolate. It is up to you to know your hot spots. I have learned that in order for me not to binge on macaroni and cheese, I can make only enough for dinner with no leftovers.

How do you handle your food drug? Do you keep lots of it around so you can tempt yourself, play tug-of-war with your mind, lose the battle and in the end beat yourself up? Or do you limit the amount you have in your home? When we know what that drug is we can face up to the why and take care of our needs in another way. If we don't, we will overdose every single time we are around it.

Most of us have eaten several times already today and we may not even have realized it. We medicate ourselves with food without a thought as to what is going into our mouth and how it will affect our body. This type of mindless eating has a way of creeping up on us while we are cooking dinner, grazing at a buffet line, or cleaning off our tables. I can hear you now: "One more bite won't hurt anything."

Not all mindless eating is triggered by pain. Sometimes we let ourselves get too hungry and then we start eating like crazy, giving in to our cravings. First we try something salty, and then we need something sweet to cut the salt. Or we may just need something with a little texture, so we go for the crunch of a cracker or chips. Before we know it we have tasted several bites of every flavor in the pantry and nothing is doing it for us. We have to learn to be good to our body and to stop and think before we feed the feelings.

This is all about taking BabySteps toward changing negative reactions to positive actions. Listen to your body to learn the difference between emotional eating versus true hunger—do you need macaroni and cheese to fill the emotional void that you are feeling, or do you need some healthy and nourishing food for your body?

We need the three basics to live: food to eat, water to drink, and air to breathe. We also need love and relationships with other people. We have hungry hearts that long for soul con- nections. When they don't happen or when they're short-changed, we often look for a way to self-medicate the pain and disappointment. For many of us, that medication takes the form of

*Leanne*

food.

For me, it is chocolate. Creamy, delicious, never-says- no-to-me chocolate. Chocolate, particularly Cadbury choco- late, reminds me of my dad and a wonderful connection I had with him. He was a very difficult man to get close to, and the one way my father and I truly connected was with food, particularly chocolate.

The chocolate connection happened when I was about seven years old. My dad had been to England visiting family and brought back a big bar of Cadbury milk chocolate. My dad and I devoured that brick of chocolate, eating the whole thing in one sitting. I remember nothing but bliss sharing that treat with my dad. We bonded through the chocolate. To this day, any chocolate vaguely reminds me of him, but the Cad- bury is, emotionally, my drug of choice. That "daddy hole" in my heart, like an open sore that never healed, was temporar- ily filled with chocolate. I longed for a real relationship with my emotionally unavailable father. In a way, it would have been easier had he not even been around—although he was in our home, I knew he was never there for me.

As I continued to grow up, I still craved love and a relationship with my father. My chocolate urge followed me into other relationships, but there was never enough chocolate to completely take the place of my father or fill the emotional voids that I felt in other relationships. Whenever I find myself feeling unloved, not loved enough, or not loved the way I want to be, chocolate is what I reach for to fill that huge pit in my heart. Consequently, chocolate and I cannot be trusted to live together in harmony. I have to make it "gone"—no matter the amount, I will see to it that I finish off the whole thing. I sit on my chocolate addiction every day. One day, I may make peace with chocolate and not have that uncontrollable urge to consume every last molecule of its chocolicious countenance. Until then, we keep our distance.

My weight didn't become an issue until I became pregnant with my first child. Until then I was an average-weight woman, about ten pounds too heavy, who would occasionally go on a crash diet, lose a few pounds, gain them back, and then do it again. That all changed when I became pregnant.

Suddenly, the license to eat as much as I could of anything I ever wanted became the main focus of my life— that and reading every book about pregnancy and babies. I spent a ridiculous amount of time at the grocery store looking for ways to indulge myself. I ate it all—from healthy foods to out-and-out junk food. Most days I ate until I was way past full and didn't care about the consequences;

I loved the fact that there was life growing inside my tummy.

By the twenty-fourth week of my pregnancy, I had already put on twenty-five pounds. I remember making dinner for my husband and myself and being absolutely exhausted and feeling sort of cramped. My husband was in a bad mood when he came home, and I was feeling so bad it was all I could do to get dinner on the table. In the middle of a bite of spaghetti, I started crying. I was afraid to tell him what was going on—by then I was having full-on contractions and I was scared I was going to lose the baby. I finally told him, we called the doctor, and off to the hospital we went.

After the initial scare, and an overnight stay in the hospital, I went home with strict orders: bed rest for the duration of my pregnancy. Now food became all that more important and I continued to pile on the weight. I made a bond with Pepperidge Farm cookies in more ways than one—my thighs can attest to that. Finally, a week past my due date, I delivered a healthy, big 9 pounds, 13 ounces baby girl. I weighed close to two hundred pounds before she was delivered; I had gained fifty-two pounds and only my stretched-out maternity clothes fit.

So how did I console myself? I kept eating. I was ashamed of my new, larger body, and I was starving all the time because I was breast-feeding. Once again, I latched onto an excuse to overeat and emotionally hid behind the food. My consolation for not getting my body back was out-of-control eating to suppress the hurt. I didn't realize it at the time, but food became a shield for me. It kept out the pain and repelled those I wanted to leave me alone—namely, my husband. I was not interested in any intimacy during that time and I used my weight gain as part of the excuse. Subconsciously, I allowed myself to continue gaining so that he would not be interested in me intimately either. This behavior became a habit, and the weight kept creeping on and creeping on until I finally hit the plus-size clothing. Even then, I didn't stop.

I stopped abusing food when it suddenly dawned on me that the food I was using as an emotional shield didn't have the power to heal my heart. I realized, "It's only food! It's not love! It's not God!" Food seemed all-powerful only when I gave it power. I had relinquished control to food for too long. I realized that I can love myself and I can take care of myself. I decided that no chocolate, no cookies, and no milk shakes can stand in my way if I don't want them to.

## Body Clutter Mission

Open your Body Clutter Control Journal to an empty page. We are going to write. Here are some questions to get you started with your journaling:

Look back for your first memory of comfort food. Is it a certain food or any food?

What is your favorite food when you need comforting?

Now, can you look back in your past to figure out why you love it so much?

Write down your first memory of using food to comfort yourself and what was happening to you and how you felt at the time.

Just write as fast and hard as you can. The writing will help you to get it out. Don't allow your perfectionism to get you hung up on grammar, punctuation, or spelling—just write! You are the only one who is going to read this.

# 2. There Is a Cure . . .
# So Why Is It So Hard?

*Leanne*

While we prefer to call being overweight Body Clutter, we will, by no means, soft-pedal the problems associated with this very personal clutter. The medical term is obesity, and for the sake of clarity and the need to articulate the very important facts about this condition, I will call Body Clutter by its medical name in this chapter.

A recent study reports that obesity is costing Americans over 90 billion dollars a year. This is an absolutely staggering amount of money that includes not only money paid out by the afflicted themselves but also money taken as losses by employers and insurance companies. The problems associated with obesity are numerous: diabetes, heart problems, cancer, stroke, knee and joint problems are just a few. The cause of obesity is no mystery and the cure is easily defined, too. Why, then, do we struggle so much with this?

We have to look again at those 90 billion dollars a year. Obviously, there is someone making a buck off our girth. There are companies that hope and pray you will help them stay in business by buying their scams, which will not help you lose any weight whatsoever unless you are looking to lose the weight of your bank account. We are courted by the promises and "money-back guarantees" that we will succeed. In the end, we are left feeling jilted and used when the latest product that late-night television is screaming at us does not follow through on its amazing claims. We are seduced by those marketing tactics because our vulnerability is palpable. They know who we are and how to make us feel that we "need" their product so we can be that Hollywood-fantasy version of thin and beautiful. Magazines and television are also full of information and guides showing young, thin, and beautiful images to portray what we can be if only we purchase what they are selling. We are left feeling that to be part of the beautiful people we must buy into their way or we will be left behind with the feeling that we are hopeless. While we know during rational times that we are not hopeless, we have waves of insecurity that wash over us, and the diet/exercise industry is there waiting for us to climb aboard their lifeboats believing we are being rescued.

Both FlyLady and I have had extensive personal experience with this. We have each drunk ourselves silly with yucky diet concoctions and have eaten numerous diet products not fit for human consumption. We've bought loads of exercise equipment and videos, health club memberships, diet pills, books, and whatever else we were convinced would make us thin. In short, we've both done it all, and how has it helped? It hasn't—it has only produced more guilt over money spent and more clutter to fling. It's only now that we have a grip on this weight-loss thing by understanding that Body Clutter leaves when BabySteps and routines are implemented. We know that behind these practical steps is the underlying principle that we must love ourselves enough to take care of the only body we will ever be given.

Most of us have been deceived by the lies of Madison Avenue advertising hype: that beautiful is only when you are painfully young and thin (a big thank you to airbrushed thighs, wrinkles, etc.). These false gods are manufactured by big business to make you feel bad about yourself and buy their fix-it products so you, too, can join the beautiful people wannabe club.

What message does this send to our children? Why do you think eating disorders are on the rise and that normal seven-year-old girls are saying, "I need to go on a diet"? Our young girls are inundated with images of pop stars and actresses who are glamourously dressed and made up. As unrealistic or inappropriate as that may be, they want to look like them. They believe they have to make themselves over and then they, too, are sold on the quick fixes offered to all of us. This self-perpetuation of the myths that are sold to us in magazines and via other media is a problem that is giving our girls eating disorders, ruining our health, and padding the wallets of an industry that does not want you to get thin and be healthy because then it would go out of business. The truth is that you need to eat less and move more. This is doable when it's done in BabySteps and is a part of your routine.

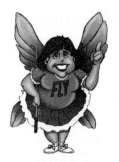

*FlyLady*

What is a diet or, for that matter, the diet industry? The word "diet" has been hijacked to become a word that has a negative meaning for most of us. What does this four-letter word really mean?

When you go back to the Greek origin of the word, *diaita*, it means "a manner of living" or *diaitasthai*, "to lead one's life." Imagine that! It is the entire way we live and the food and drink we consume to sustain our lives day in and day out. When our doctors put us on a special food regimen, it is usually to improve the quality of our "manner of living."

We have to quit feeling deprived or punished when we hear the word "diet." It is not at all about hurting ourselves; it is just about taking better care of ourselves by Finally Loving Yourself enough actually to take the BabySteps to control our behavior.

I want you to think long and hard about the diet industry. If we were all living a healthy lifestyle, would there even be one? We would naturally be eating what our body needs. This, however, is not the case. Instead we overeat and then look for the instant cure that is going to make those unwanted pounds vanish. It is our desire for a quick fix that has allowed the diet industry to flourish into the 42-billion-dollar business that it is today. And that is just the diet industry itself; it does not include the 90 billion dollars a year that is spent on the health-related issues of obesity that Leanne referred to. This means that the cost of obesity and trying to fight it is well over 130 billion dollars a year!

This industry is made up of pills, vitamins, exercise equipment, videos, gym memberships, food club memberships, and books. We hope that this book is the last book you ever have to buy! Our goal is to teach you about your body and the clutter that has collected in your head, on your thighs, and in your pantry. We want to give you a new attitude about your body and a new perspective when it comes to the food you consume. These changes do not happen overnight. They are a series of BabySteps that you take to help you climb the staircase of success in finding a new way of living.

When I first started to attempt to get my home in order, I looked at several different self-help books in bookstores and I even bought a few; my attempts were almost always a failure. My ventures into weight-loss land have been even more involved than all of those get-organized-now or get-rich-quick schemes we have all fallen victim to at one time or another. I will start by naming them in the order that I tried them, beginning in 1974.

1. Water pills (fainted)
2. Diet pills (got really fussy)
3. The Cabbage Soup Diet (I think it was Dolly Parton's recipe—got sick of it)

4. Started jogging (badgered into this by ex-husband; made my shins hurt)
5. Special dehydrated food, a membership, and meetings (bought all the food and never went back)
6. Read the book *Overcoming Overeating* (made sense)
7. Overeaters Anonymous (one meeting—made a lot of sense!)
8. Took aerobics class (I am aerobically challenged)
9. Weight Watchers (joined several times, went once and never went back)
10. Joined a gym (yes, I went once)
11. Bought video workout tapes (never played them)
12. Bought a video for tai chi (watched once)
13. Bought several books on tai chi (never opened them)
14. Bought a Richard Simmons video (did it five times)
15. Read *The Weigh Down Diet* (gave several away)
16. Joined Weigh Down Diet Program (went three times)
17. Read the book *Thin Within* (made a lot more sense)
18. Bought a book about reducing carb intake (don't even know the name—gave it away)
19. Bought a treadmill (the only thing I have ever stuck with because I can write while doing it)
20. Read a book about eating for your blood type (interesting idea)

Do you see a pattern here? I like to call it the "magic pill syndrome." We buy it and think it is going to be the quick fix to our battle of the bulge. We do it for a short while, and then we never do it again. Why? All I can figure out is that any and all of these different ways will work if you use them. If you don't, they won't. Why couldn't I use them? What got in my way? Was it my own perfectionism? Or perhaps it was my rebellious spirit—more of the clutter I needed to get rid of from a bad marriage. No one was going to make me feel bad again. I love me just the way I am.

Here is the hard part—I really do love me! If I hadn't let go of all that guilt and self-loathing I would have continued to gain weight. Or could it just be that the person who filled my head with ugliness was no longer in my life and that lack of stress caused me to quit gaining weight? I don't know and it really doesn't matter! The most important thing I had to keep in the front of my mind was loving myself enough to want to live a long and healthy life—and that I am not now, and will never be, the next supermodel or cover girl. But I can love myself just for being me.

I have been FLYing for several years now. It took me nine months to get rid of the clutter in our home. The clutter went away with the help of *27-Fling Boogies, HotSpot Fire Drills,* and *5-Minute Room Rescues.* All the while my timer was keeping me focused! In our all-or-nothing thinking we would love to crisis-clean our thighs and not wait for the results of the slow and steady process of changing our lifestyle. Let's be realistic here. The clutter in our home didn't happen in a week, or a month or even a year. It is a collection that grew and grew our whole lives.

Our bodies are like our homes. In fact the body is the home of our soul, the temple of our being. If we would just be as careful about what we put in our body as we are about what

we bring into our home, then we would have an amazing attitude shift. Someone once told me, "You are what you eat and if
you eat fat you will be fat." For some reason that has always
stuck with me—not that I used to pay much attention to it. I
have become more particular about what I put in my
body/temple. It is the only one I have and it is worth taking
care of. I teach others how to declutter their homes by having
them look at each thing and asking some tough questions:

Do I love you?

Do you make me smile?

Do I have a place for you?

If the answer is no—out you go!

How can we use this same approach to the food we put in
our mouth? If we ask ourselves, "Do I love you?" to chocolate
or chips, we will say, "Why, of course!" Gobble, gobble and
they will be gone. "Do you make me smile?" "Yes, sir, with
every single bite." "Do I have a place for you?" "Yes I do, right
in my tummy!" But the truth is where it will really go—right
on your thighs or your Franny.

Let's look at some questions we can ask the food as we
take a bite:

Are you going to bless my body?

Do you fit into my healthy way of eating?

Is your taste worthy enough to go into my body?

Why do I want to eat you?

**Are you going to bless my body?** With the first question we are looking for good nutrition: vitamins, minerals,
fiber, and protein.

**Do you fit into my healthy way of eating?** This one is a simple yes or no.

**Is your taste worthy enough to go into my body?** If something has no taste, why would you want to put it in your body? Hey, I am telling you this because in the past I have pigged out on rice cakes. Why? That is our next question.

**Why do I want to eat you?** Am I really hungry, or do I just need a drink of water? Am I angry and want to eat to stuff my feelings? Am I lonely and feeling sorry for myself, or am I just tired and really need to go to bed? Is this mindless eating? HALT and think about it for a second. HALT stands for: Hungry, Angry, Lonely, or Tired.

There is balance in all things, from TV watching to eating. We all have to find our own balance, what fits us as individuals. I do know that this is not rocket science; it is really just plain common sense, but we have to think just a little before we bite.

For seventeen years I was married to my first husband and father of my only child. At best, it was a stressful period of my life, and I kept my feelings stuffed down most of the time. When I left, I started FLYing for the first time. I worked hard at learning to love myself—I had to get rid of the constant brainwashing that told me that I was incompetent, ugly, and fat, and that I was nothing and never would be anything. I had to turn those words around and have them bless me. No one else was going to do it for me; I had to do this one by myself. I now know why I had to go through all of this—I could not help you if I had not!

I recently realized that I still have two things from that other life that are with me daily. One is good and the other could still hurt me if I didn't deal with it. The wonderful gift I have is my son. I am very thankful for him. The negative thing is my weight. I am well aware of the health risks of being overweight and that is where loving myself has come into my life. I am working on becoming healthier so that I can live in peace and joy for a long time. In spite of being overweight, I have learned to love me as I am and not to beat myself up anymore. I am now taking the BabySteps that I need to allow me to live the life I was meant to live. My body is the temple that I live in and should never be despised or disrespected.

My sister Paddi and I thought that when I met Robert, my Sweet Darling, the weight would just fall right off me, but it has not. We thought that because I was happier, those years of clutter would just disappear, but that has not happened either. I collected this clutter a long time ago and it is going to take more than wishing and happiness to make it go away. I always say, "You can't organize clutter, you can only get rid of it." I have been the same size for many years. I stopped adding Body Clutter and only recently have started getting rid of it. The question that you have to ask yourself is, "How do I deal with the issue of being overweight and what could it do to my health and my happy life?"

BabySteps and routines are the cure for clutter in your home. Body Clutter, too, has a cure, and with BabySteps and routines we can live healthier, happier, longer lives. Finally Loving Yourself is not about being magazine-cover thin and perfect. It is about loving yourself enough to be as healthy as you can be for you and, in turn, for those you love.

## Body Clutter Mission

It is time to open up your Body Clutter Control Journal. When you get your feelings out of you and on paper, you won't have to hold them inside any longer. Do not allow your perfectionism to stop you on your journey. This is not about the color ink you are using or your punctuation. Just write!

What is your image of beautiful?

Write down the list of diet schemes that you have tried and put down how you did with them and what you felt about them.

Next, go back to your teenage years and write down what you remember about your weight. You can reconstruct your life according to what you weighed when something big happened in your life: graduation, marriage, birth, moving, promotion, etc. If you have "weight amnesia," then write what you can remember. When you have finished, try to associate the areas of weight gain to what was going on in your life.

Do you have any health issues related to your weight? Diabetes, joint problems, foot problems, or anything else you can think of?

# 3. The Hidden, and Not So Hidden, Realities of Body Clutter

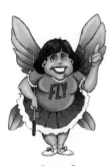

*FlyLady*

There is a hidden agenda behind Body Clutter and we have developed strategies for hiding it from ourselves. We're running and ducking and looking for cover, and we don't even realize that who we're really running from is ourselves.

We start by trying to hide our weight—from living in a muumuu to out-and-out denial. If we can fool ourselves into thinking that it's not showing, then we can pretend it's not there and continue in our self-fulfilling prophecy that we will always be stuck with Body Clutter. The fat clothes/skinny clothes taking up room in our closets, the great big sweaters and looking forward to winter so we can cover up all go back to the same thing—we're hiding.

## Fat Clothes/Skinny Clothes

We play a game that is a form of torture and self-punishment: reminding ourselves that we've "failed" to live up to our narrow, idealistic vision of who we once were and who we would like to be again.

But try as we may to hide behind the big clothes, our skinny clothes are standing by, reaching out to us in the closet, silent witnesses to the fact that our bottom is bigger and rounder. Although we know better, we still hang on to those guilt-producing garments. We can't help but beat ourselves up just one more time. Most of us have skinny clothes that are out of style and even all wrong for us in our current lifestyles. If we're going to be new creations by attempting to redefine ourselves and change, well, then, those clothes must go. You can't organize clutter; you can only get rid of it.

## "I Feel Pretty"

We have all heard this song and right now you need to take a minute and ask yourself, "Do I feel pretty?" If your answer is NO! then here is your first assignment: When you join FlyLady, the first thing we ask you to do each day is get up and get dressed to shoes and fix your hair and face so you can greet the day ready to confront anything or anyone! Are you doing this? If not, why are you refusing this one simple request?

I can hear you now, "I don't feel this is necessary, because I am not going to see anyone today but my babies." This kind of thinking is just another excuse. All I want is for you to smile when you see yourself in the mirror. Can you do that with chicken hair sticking up all over your head? You may be able to belly-laugh, but can you look in the mirror and feel good about what you see? Do you feel pretty?

Feeling pretty is more about your attitude than your face. Sometimes our attitudes need a little help. I know many of you think that getting dressed is not important for keeping your home in order and getting rid of Body Clutter, but I want you to do this for me at first if you can't bring yourself to do it just for you. My Granny always said, "Pretty is as pretty does!" As a child I had interpreted that to mean if you act right you will be considered pretty. Now that I am grown up and I have finally started to love myself, I can see a whole new beautiful meaning to this unwritten law: If you don't treat yourself with respect and love, you will not feel pretty. Getting up and taking care of you is the most important job of your whole day. Lying around in your jammies all day does not make you feel pretty. So in order to feel pretty you have to do something about your appearance. Your fairy godmother is not going to wave a magic wand over you and turn you into a princess. Bibbity, Bobbity, Boo!

We have all had those mornings when we didn't feel it was necessary to get prettied up. Now that I have been doing my Morning Routine for several years, it is next to impossible for me not to get dressed to shoes. Even when I am sick, I always get dressed to shoes.

Now I want to talk about what clothes we put on. Do your clothes make you feel ugly? Are they too tight because you have gained a few extra pounds? Are you holding on to your skinny clothes in hope that you will lose the weight one day? In the meantime you are beating yourself up over the fact that you can't wear that one outfit that made you feel like a million bucks. That outfit yells at you each time you open your closet door. Get rid of loud, ill-tempered clothing! Don't keep anything in your home that makes you have bad feelings. This has got to stop! It doesn't matter for now if you have only one everyday outfit that you feel pretty in.

I don't want you wearing clothes that are too big, either! Frumpy sweats have a way of telling our head that it is okay to eat that extra cookie, because no one will notice anyway. Before you know it, you will be filling out those baggy sweatpants. Any of us can look pretty and feel cute in a pair of jeans and a shirt. It is all a state of mind and having clothes that fit you properly. When you love yourself enough to wear only things that make you feel good about yourself, then you will not torture your body with clothes that are too tight or too baggy.

The idea of feeling pretty also has to do with your underclothes, favorite pieces of jewelry, a special color of lipstick, or even a sweet-smelling bath bar. It all comes down to your attitude. Love yourself by just being nice to you. "Pretty is as pretty does."

This morning I blow-dried my hair. I hardly ever do this, but a little poof makes me feel special, as does an evening bubble bath and a morning shower. Try it some-time. You are worth it. Now don't complain that you are too heavy to feel pretty. That outlook is all wrong. Pretty has nothing to do with your weight! I feel pretty and I am not a size ten.

In a picture of me in a women's magazine, I had on my favorite denim jumper and a red shirt. I like red; I feel powerful in red. I am even wearing red right this minute. In red I feel "pretty and witty and wise!" We know the song. Start singing and have fun feeling pretty. You are FLYing when you feel pretty!

## The Hidden Realities of Body Clutter

The not-so-hidden realities of Body Clutter are what we have just covered: the hiding behind the big clothing, the excuses, and the thoughts that we are not worthy of feel-ing pretty. We are now going to uncover the hidden real-ities of Body Clutter.

As we were working on this book, the one thing that was a constant for us was to be as honest with you, the reader, as we possibly could. Ouch! This means actually recognizing some very painful things about our bodies and how we are affected by Body Clutter.

We can cover up our Body Clutter with clothing that is baggy or even with clothing that fits well, just like we hide our household clutter in pretty boxes and plastic tubs. But we are all faced with the truth when we take off our clothes in the bathroom to get in the tub or shower. That is when we can no longer lie to ourselves. Our mirrors are brutal, but the voices in our head are sometimes much worse than the eyeful we refuse to look at in the light of day.

Right now I want to discuss the things that we usually do not talk about in public—the physical reality of our Body Clutter. I will never forget the first time I leaned against my washer and felt a pinch. My little roll of fat had become a big roll and it hurt when I reached into my washer to pull out the wet clothes. There are many other painful moments when it comes to Body Clutter.

Let's think about what happens in the privacy of our bathroom. There is no worse feeling than sitting in a tub or standing in a shower that is too small for us. Then there is the problem of actually sitting down in the tub— it is more like falling into it, and getting out of it is often more difficult than getting in. There is also the claustrophobic feeling when standing in a shower stall that feels like the walls are closing in on you. We could go on and on. Here's another example: How about covering up with a mound of bubbles in the tub and turning the lights down low so you really don't have to look at yourself? Bubble baths, which can be lovely, should be used for comfort and relaxation, not for hiding from yourself.

Then there are the issues of personal hygiene. I know this isn't a pretty picture, but we all have to sit on the "throne" every day. It is a fact of life: When your Body Clutter gets in the way of doing this efficiently, it can be painful in more ways than your ego getting hurt.

Now what about summertime? We all love summer and fun summer clothes. Summer is painful. There are rashes and raw places that happen when certain body parts rub together. You know, the rolls of fat, our under-arms, and everyone's favorite—our thunder thighs. We even quit wearing sleeveless dresses and tops because of the way our arms look. Shorts are a thing of the past be-cause they ride up on the thighs and we have to keep pulling them down from their wedgie position. Cool sum-mer dresses seem appealing and almost an answer to the sleeveless shirt and shorts problem, but the thighs rub to-gether, then the heat rash begins, and soon we become raw in places that will hurt all summer long.

Although I said we were going to be honest, I am not even going to discuss putting on a bathing suit; it has been so long since some of us wore one that we have for-gotten how it feels or all the prep work that needs to be done before you put one on. I had a friend remind me about trying to shave "that" area and how difficult it was when you can't even see down there. No bathing suit equals no swimming, which can be a great and gentle way to move our body. Do you see how these physical limita-tions keep us sedentary? We are so tired, tired of not feel-ing like we can do anything. It is time that we start living again!

Winter is another story. At least we can put on enough clothes to cover up and protect our thighs, but try wear-ing corduroy pants and listen to the awful serenade while you walk. Buying clothes, especially panty hose, is tough—when you find a pair that fits your belly and thighs, then it bags at the ankles. They cost us a small fortune, too, and all for one wear, because once we take them off, we find the thighs have holes rubbed in them.

Boots are fun winter clothes, but not for people who have big calves. Have you ever shopped for boots? Not an enjoyable experience. Then when you finally find a pair that fits, you need someone to help you get them off. I guess that is why slouch boots were invented. Another problem is tying our shoes. We have to grab our pant leg to pull our foot close enough to fasten it.

Let's discuss what the extra weight does to our legs and feet. When you are carrying around a lot of Body Clutter, your shoes wear out faster, not the outside but the cushions on the inside. We need really good shoes with great support and they cost some money. I have found if I don't wear good shoes that are new and made for big people, then my heel or Achilles tendon hurts and I have trouble walking—another way that my weight adds to my sedentary lifestyle.

Then we have our bosoms. We try to support them with the over-the-shoulder-boulder-holders just so we will not rub raw places below them. We have a hard time sleeping because they are in our way—sleeping on our tummy is gone forever, as if our belly didn't already get in the way. The weight of our breasts causes our bra straps to dig into our shoulders, resulting in shoulder problems and nerve damage.

Our extra weight hurts our joints, muscles, bones, and skin. The more Body Clutter we have, the less we want to move, and the less we move, the more clutter we collect. It is one enormous vicious cycle.

Now let's look at the embarrassment we feel because of our size. Yes, we already know how hard it is to get around and how winded we get from just moving. But now I want to talk about those seat belts in the backseat of the car that don't go around us or having to ask someone else to fasten it for you because you can't reach it. There have been times that I have not wanted to fasten it because of how humiliated I feel. How sad is it that I could be risking my life because of my shame?

Then there is the pain of not fitting in a booth at a restaurant or a movie theater seat. At least in the dark theater our shame is hidden. What about not being able to cross your legs? Another area of pain is when we have to travel. Airplane seats are small and uncomfortable to begin with, and no one wants to ask for the belt extender. Let's face it—our size gets in the way of having fun.

This is not easy to talk about, but I am determined to discuss these things so you will know that you are not alone. Many of us suffer silently with pain and embarrassment. I just want you to know that my heart goes out to you. Writing this has been very difficult and I am sure for some of you very hard to read. This is where FLYing is so important. Finally Loving Yourself. Loving yourself enough to be able to see and deal with the realities of who and what we are and what we can be—healthier and happier for the rest of our lives.

FlyLady has spoken openly about the hidden, and not so hidden, realities of Body Clutter. She mentioned stuff no one has ever had the guts to talk about—the secret stuff we have kept to ourselves.

*Leanne*

She also talked about hiding behind the big clothing and not feeling pretty. My story is slightly different. In a way, I welcomed the Body Clutter into my life and the truth is I purposely gained weight to keep my (now ex) husband away from me. I didn't know that at the time, of course. Today I not only know this to be true, but I understand why.

I was married to my ex-husband for nearly seventeen years. It most definitely wasn't a match made in heaven. I was very unhappy in the relationship and it showed up on my body. I weighed 125 pounds when we married, and by the time we separated (for the third and final time), I weighed 200 pounds.

For the three months following the final separation, I went through the most stress I've ever experienced in my life, including full-blown panic attacks. I wasn't sleeping well, could hardly eat, and jumped if the phone rang. I put on 10 pounds a month those three months, kicking my weight up to a grand total of 230 pounds. The truth of the matter is I had gained well over 100 pounds in seventeen years of marriage. That was when I found out my

thyroid wasn't working as it should and was put on medication. After doing a lot of reading and research, I found
some interesting information from a holistic point of view:
The thyroid gland itself reflects a woman's voice in her
life. Unresolved conflict and stress can rob a woman of
her voice and, consequently, it's as if her voice becomes
"trapped." I know that sounds bizarre, but I also knew
that for me the truth was undeniable. I had lost my voice
in my life and the control that went with it many years
before. And my thyroid gland was reflecting that by not
working properly.

But back to the marriage itself. There were highlights.
Their names are Caroline and Peter, and the best days of
my marriage were the days when my children were born.
Four years into our marriage, I had my children pretty
much back to back—two babies in less than two years.
Think about this for a minute . . . a very unhappy marriage plus two babies. Double diapers, double stroller,
double car seats—are you feeling the pain yet?

They were both big babies at birth, one nearly ten
pounds, and the other well over nine pounds. I had gained
fifty-two pounds with my first pregnancy due to prema-
ture labor and needing to adhere to the doctor's advice
regarding bed rest starting in the 24th week. Let's not forget that I also consumed way too much food and developed an overt fondness for Pepperidge Farm cookies. My
firstborn ended up being late and I was induced, produc-
ing the nearly ten-pound Caroline!

With the second pregnancy, I walked three miles a day,

was careful about my diet, and gained only twenty-seven pounds. The problem was that the weight from the first pregnancy hadn't all come off yet, and when I learned I was pregnant with number two, I was still several pounds overweight. After a year of nursing my second baby, I tried again to implement the walking/dieting regimen I had started with my second pregnancy and finally got down to 165 pounds. I was beginning to feel better about myself.

Unfortunately, that's when things really started to go downhill with my marriage. I've learned since then that in a dysfunctional marriage, when one spouse starts to feel better about himself or herself, the other one steps up the dysfunctional behavior. I was intimidated by my husband and at times scared. To protect myself and to keep him away, I started overeating (I especially abused chocolate), quit exercising, and built myself a "suit of armor": my own personal Body Clutter protection kit. If I couldn't leave the marriage (I was too scared), then I might as well protect myself as best I could. And let's face it, if you don't look good, you're less likely to have an amorous spouse. Well, sort of. Maybe his advances slowed down, but they never completely went away and I absolutely dreaded them. The fact was that our relationship was such a shambles that it made something that should be beautiful between a husband and wife completely worthless.

But I kept up appearances and just bought bigger clothes. I lied to myself about what was going on in my life and with my marriage (and the residual effect of putting on the Body Clutter) because the truth was too painful to see. The funny thing is that once I started telling the truth, I became empowered—incrementally, for sure, and definitely not all at once. But the point was, I wasn't powerless anymore. Little did I know the journey I was about to embark on!

I knew and understood the biblical principles of reaping and sowing. But I didn't understand the biblical principle of doing unto myself as I did unto others. Yeah, okay, so it's a little in reverse. I think that's because the writer of those words of wisdom assumed you loved yourself! Think about this for a minute . . . you cannot give to others something you don't have, and if you don't have love for yourself, how then can you truly love others? I think you can feel the emotion of love and go through the motions, but you cannot truly experience it in the depth of your soul and really live it until you love yourself first. Whew, that was a biggie for me, and the beginning of my own personal transformation of both body and soul.

One of the things that hit me was that my happiness was not built on other people, my marriage, a dress size, or my assessment of how my children were doing. In my perfectionism, I tried hard to base my happiness quotient on all of those things and was in utter despair because in my eyes I was a complete failure. My marriage was a sham—those closest to me knew it and the "other people," for whom I put on my dog-and-pony show, hardly knew my name, let alone what the heck was going on in my life. Looking back, I think it's hilarious that I was so wrapped up in what "other people" thought.

The point is, I moved my assessment of what constituted personal happiness away from being dependent on people, places, or things. In doing so, I moved beyond the garbage that was holding me back so I could finally find happiness. My marriage was over way before I left, but physically leaving was the next thing.

The last item on the list was to deal with my Body Clutter. But in order to deal with it, I needed to accept myself *first* as I was. I had to buy clothes in the plus-size stores. I was unhappy that I had to shop there, but I made peace with my size and with my body. Right then, my only goal was to dress to look nice. To me, that was the ultimate unveiling of who I was. I was a larger woman, but I was still me deep down inside and I just needed to love me for who I was. So you know what? I did! And the result of accepting my (tight) size-eighteen self was the opening of a new era for wanting to take care of myself even more, and eventually I started wholeheartedly, truly loving myself and taking the BabySteps I needed to take to begin losing the Body Clutter that I had used for so many years as a shield. I didn't need that kind of protection anymore. It was time for it to go.

## Body Clutter Mission

As you go through each chapter of this book, take a few moments to reflect on what you have read.

Do you feel pretty? If you answer no, then write about how you feel about the way you look. Two things to remember: No one is going to read this and you are not allowed to be mean to yourself. Do not allow your perfectionism to keep you from your journey to discover the Body Clutter you have hiding deep inside you.

How many years' worth of clothes do you have in your closet? And, better yet, how many sizes? What words do you hear in your head when you look in your closet at the clothes that don't fit?

Do you get dressed to shoes first thing in the morning?

Have you ever felt embarrassed by your weight? Write about how you felt and what caused your shame.

Have you used your Body Clutter as a shield? In what way and who or what were you trying to protect yourself from?

# 4. Excuses, Excuses!

Oprah Winfrey once said, "Real integrity is doing the right thing, knowing that nobody's going to know whether you did it or not." I have a real admiration for Oprah Winfrey. She might not be everyone's cup of tea, but I admire her ability to cut to the chase and get right to the heart of the matter. And for someone who has battled her Body Clutter in a very public arena, that quote brings to mind some very important issues as we struggle with our own Body Clutter.

*Leanne*

Excuses—the lies we tell ourselves and others to get them on "our side." We want people to understand that our Body Clutter isn't our fault because we are "victims." My favorite one was blaming my thyroid. Well, yeah, thyroid conditions can make Body Clutter loss hard, but not impossible. It means you have to work with your doctor to get your medication right and you have to work your Franny off at the gym making sure you get the exercise that is critical in dumping the pounds. The fact of the matter is (and brace yourself, this is going to hurt) that our excuses reveal a lack of character on our part, an ugly dent in our personal integrity. Doing the right thing means you do it when no one is looking and you do it for the right reasons. It's just that simple.

There are a bazillion and one excuses out there for not taking care of your Body Clutter. I've used most of them and so have you. The minute I got serious about my Body Clutter, I recognized those excuses for what they were: character flaws that exposed a serious deficit in my own personal integrity. That revelation was completely devastating. But do you know what? We are the biggest deceivers on the planet when it comes to ourselves.

How many times have you said, "On Monday, I'm going to (fill in the blank)"? For me that blank was: get serious, start exercising, eat right, etc. And as Monday came and went, nine times out of ten I didn't start, and even those rare times I did, my good intentions were dashed against the rocks by Wednesday.

But I learned some things along the way and, thank God, I never gave up. Like FlyLady says, jump in where you are! It really doesn't matter how many pounds of Body Clutter you need to declutter, the fact is there is work to be done. When you begin to understand, like Fly-

Lady and I did, that paying attention to your fuel and movement isn't just so that you can wear a smaller size, but it is critical for doing more of the work that God had called us to do. It isn't just vanity, but it is a whole new life that God wanted to reveal to us.

Here's something that totally blew me away: Perfectionism is also evident in staying where you are. Listen to this—FlyLady and I both did this. We always say you must accept yourself first as you are today before you can work on your Body Clutter. That is very true. However, the kicker is staying there. FlyLady has said, "My weight hasn't changed in fifteen years." That is an excuse *and* perfectionism because, by saying that, she is really saying, "I'm not willing to change." And being unwilling to change is simply another way of being paralyzed by perfectionism, because if you can't do it right, you're not going to do it all. Then what follows are the excuses and rationalizations.

We're all intelligent enough people. We somehow manage to run households, raise children, hold jobs, and yet we search for the elusive "fix" for our weight problem. If our children were to come to us with a math problem they couldn't figure out, we'd sit down with them and explain the steps. We would show them why they needed to take *each* step in the correct order to solve the math problem.

Our weight issues are exactly the same. As much as we want the magic-wand approach (much like our children do when trying to get their math homework done), we know intuitively and intellectually that it is truly a logical issue that requires one small BabyStep at a time. Why then do we fight this truth so hard?

It seems to me that our excuses insulate us from the facts. In other words, if we can rally behind the rationalizations, we are home free—or so we think. We don't have to face the music then. Our clothing size continues to get larger and, consequently, health problems continue to mount. We look for miracle cures for our new aches and pains without taking into account the obvious—we need to lose the Body Clutter!

It was Ann Landers who made "Wake up and smell the coffee" the popular phrase it is today. I've thought a lot about this and how we miss the most obvious things and why we won't step up and accept the truth. There is a lot of pain associated with honesty, but there is also tremendous freedom that comes the moment the lights go on. And to me, the fact that you are reading this is a golden opportunity for you to become gut honest with yourself and get real with what your excuses truly are about your own Body Clutter. You want to and can do *something*, otherwise you never would have picked up this book in the first place! Start with the Body Clutter between your ears—get real, get honest, and face it. Scary proposition, yes, but only for a moment! Then you have the opportunity to savor the victory—the first BabyStep to freedom from Body Clutter.

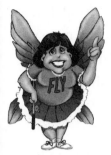

*FlyLady*

When and why did we start believing all the lies we told ourselves? All those excuses we made up to justify our Body Clutter? This is perfectionism, plain and simple, and at its ugliest. It was easier to tell ourselves a lie than it was to accept that we were not perfect.

Deep in our hearts we know that we are not perfect and we don't have to be, but that doesn't stop the pursuit of perfectionism. It doesn't even occur to us that is what we are doing; it just becomes accepted behavior that excuses are the way we deal with our refusal to get rid of our Body Clutter. The lies make it easier for us to pretend to love ourselves, but they only end up creating even more Body Cutter. It becomes a vicious cycle of lying to ourselves and stuffing our face to push down the guilt.

Think about the women who suffer from eating disorders. When we see pictures of them, we don't see what they see in themselves. They see imperfection. When we look at ourselves, we see imperfections, too. That is why we try to make ourselves believe the lies. Both perspectives are lies that cause harm to our bodies.

Another way to look at this is through my FlyLady eyes. There is not much difference between a born-organized person and a sidetracked person—the dividing line is perfectionism. The born-organized person goes over the line with her cleaning while the sidetracked person gets up to that same line and backs away. She doesn't have time to do it right, so why even bother? What does she do at this time but start making the same old excuses for her messy house? We have all resorted to those excuses and we know what they are. We are just trying with some fresh paint to gloss over the real truth that would make us look bad. All the lies do is fill us with even more guilt.

Our bodies are just like our homes. As we kept trying to fill that empty hole in our hearts with stuff, we were also turning to food for comfort. We don't like looking at this, but the truth is that we don't want to face the reality that we are not, and will never be, perfect. So instead of saying, "Why bother?" unconsciously we made up lies to make ourselves more lovable. Who are we lying to? No one really believes us. It may help us feel better for a little while, but in the long run we have blinded ourselves to the reality of what Body Clutter actually does to us.

Body Clutter destroys our life! It robs us of our days on this earth. What days we do have are filled with pain and sickness. We may not want to look at this without our rose-colored glasses, but ask yourself, have you ever seen a one-hundred-year-old fat person? Until recently, our society has been living longer than any previous generation. However, obesity is the cause of many of our health problems and is now lowering life-expectancy figures. Right now I am dealing with diabetes. If that doesn't make you take off your rose-colored glasses, then just read a few of the health complications associated with diabetes.

Let's just start with vision problems. That was when I got my first diagnosis of a potential problem with my blood sugar levels. My eye doctor saw something while examining my eyes that concerned him and told me to go get a test for diabetes. I made an appointment for a wellness check. That was about all I did. They drew blood and I got the report that my sugar level was a little high but I still had on my rose-colored glasses and decided that I would just stop drinking my sweet tea and colas. That decreased my other symptoms of increased thirst and frequent urination in the middle of the night. I had thought that my toothpaste was causing my thirst problem. Those rose-colored glasses can really blind us when we don't address our health problems. Diabetes eventually robs us of our sight. Just because we don't think it will happen to us does not mean we are protected. Let's not fool ourselves—we deserve honesty.

Then there is an increased risk of heart and circulatory problems. Oh, and let's not forget about kidney failure. Since I have been struggling with my Body Clutter . . . no, let's call a spade a spade! Since I have been overweight for the last thirty years, my body and my health have been telling me to change my bad, ineffective ways of addressing my weight and lack of exercise. My body has been yelling at me, "I want to live and be healthy! Why are you ignoring me?" It tells me this every time I am unable to walk up a flight of stairs, sit in a chair comfortably, or take a walk with my husband. My fat is making me miss out on living.

Along with all the excuses that keep us from ever addressing our obesity, we also have fear. So we make up a whole new set of lies to cover up how scared we really are of change. At least our fat is familiar. But we picture those images of so-called thin and beautiful people, and we want to change and vow to diet. Then we think, "What if I fail? Oh, and what if I succeed?!" We beat ourselves up before we ever get started. No wonder we are afraid! We are the worst abuser of all—we abuse ourselves. We are afraid even to try, so we have fooled ourselves into believing we are just fine the way we are. Well, a 252-pound woman is not healthy even if her blood pressure is good and her cholesterol is low. We allow our perfectionism to hurt us once again.

What are we doing when we hide in the car and scarf down doughnuts or a big greasy burger and french fries? Who are we kidding? No wonder we can't lose weight; we don't really want it bad enough. We set ourselves up for failure because we are dishonest with the most important person in the world. If we can't tell ourselves the truth, then what have we come to? I know you want to curl up in a ball right now and feel sorry for yourself, but that is what this kind of sneak eating is all about—feeling sorry for yourself.

Losing weight is not a game we play. It is not a challenge we take on to beat someone by losing more weight than she can. This is a lifelong attitude adjustment. It is okay that we are just now making the decision to change. We can jump in right where we are and not look back, but only look forward. This is not the hard work you have forced yourself to believe it is; wellness is a choice to live a balanced life. It's not work unless we make it that way. An example of this is emptying the dishwasher. It takes only a few minutes, but we keep ourselves from actually doing it because we are too busy complaining and thinking about how long it will take. Work is what we call it when it seems too hard to do and we don't want to do it. When you catch yourself rebelling against starting a new habit because you think it is going to be too hard, I want you to hear those lies you are telling yourself. Let me tell you what is really hard—not taking the necessary BabySteps to regain your health, and that is what will keep you from living an active life. By active all I mean is being able to climb a flight of stairs or get out of your car. Not being able to play with your babies or leaving your spouse to spend his life alone—now that is hard.

Let's think about why we have failed in the past to establish any new habits. Most of the time we go hog-wild at first and try to do too much too fast. We all know what happens next. We crash and burn. I want us to back up to why we decided to start a new habit in the first place.

If you are not doing it for you, then it is a given that you are going to fail. So many times we do things for our husbands, children, and parents. We have done things for people we don't even know. This may sound a bit obscure, but I want you to think about external gratification. When we do things to win the adoration of others, we are not doing it for ourselves. This is just another lie we believe. For a new habit to become automatic, we have to cheer ourselves on and not depend on the feelings or words from others.

When you find a vocation that you love, as I have, you can work many hours a day and it doesn't even seem like work, which is what has happened to me with my lifestyle change. It is a labor of love to bless my life with a healthy body. The Body Clutter I have lost is just a side effect of my healthy-eating BabySteps. My goal was not weight loss, it was to live a healthier life. I realized a long time ago that I could not change too many things at once. That is how BabySteps have changed my home, my mind, and now my health—one small step at a time.

BabySteps are just subtle changes in our attitudes that we turn into simple actions that we practice daily. They are going to help you more than anything else you can do for yourself. It is all about being kind to yourself and not piling on more than you can do.

**Excuses! Excuses! Excuses!**
We have all made them and we will continue to make them until we wake up and recognize that these excuses are part of that alternate reality (Body Clutter) that we are hiding in.

Here are the excuses we tell ourselves and others to keep us secure in our Body Clutter!

❂ **I am just big boned!** Yeah, right! The length of our bones makes us tall; they may even be big around, but it is the fat we have on our bodies that puts the weight on our skeleton. We use this as one of most common excuses to make us feel better. But does it really?

❂ **Everyone in my family is big; it must just be heredity.** Well, the truth for me is that I have two sisters and a grandmother who are petite. So what is really my problem? Excuses are just a category of lies.

❁ **I have a slow metabolism.** This one may actually be true. Our metabolism slows down because we starve our body by not eating healthfully. Our body fears there is a lack of food, a famine, so it goes into preservation mode to reserve our body fat for those days without food. When are we going to start treating ourselves better by eating regularly and putting good fuel in our body?

❁ **I can't afford diet food/healthy food.** So how much do your doctor bills cost you? Eating well doesn't cost much when you plan your meals. Special diet food is not anything you can live with for a lifetime.

❁ **I don't have time to cook two meals—one for me and one for my family.** Of course you don't, and you don't have to. Feeding your family nutritious, wholesome food is good for you and for them. Only one meal is all you need to fix.

❁ **I am just getting older—you know, the middle-age spread.** If that is the case, then middle age for me started at the age of twenty and I should be dead by now.

❁ **I have had children—I was eating for two.** Those precious little packages that weighed less than ten pounds! The one truth here is we took those nine months to start excess-eating habits and kept right on after the baby was born.

✿ **I quit smoking and that's why I put on this weight.** I applaud you for stopping smoking. Bad habits are hard to break. So naturally you reached for food to put something in your hand and then into your mouth. It is not a good idea to replace one bad habit with another—mindless eating. And please don't use weight gain as an excuse not to quit smoking!

✿ **Why even bother to try to lose? I can't do it.** Here you go again, putting yourself down before you even start! This is our perfectionism rearing its ugly head again! The reason you have not been able to lose weight and keep it off is that you have never taken BabySteps to do it! Be kind to yourself and establish good eating habits and a simple exercise routine to help you get healthier.

✿ **I am happy with me just the way I am.** Oh, how many times I have said this one, not to mention the number of times I have put it in writing to you! "Where ignorance is bliss, 'tis folly to be wise" (Thomas Gray). I have wised up now to my personal deception. It is not a happy person who mistreats the only body she has by not eating well.

✿ **If I lost weight, I couldn't afford to buy new clothes.** Oh, poor you! Excuses are such a wasted use of words! If the truth be known, you probably still have some of your skinny clothes in your closet. You are not going to go naked. The money you save by not eating fast food each week can buy you a new pair of jeans.

❂ **My weight protects me from unwanted attention.** It keeps my husband at a distance and it also protects me from other men who may be attracted to me. That is not what the weight is doing. You are doing this by your own lack of self-love. If you don't take care of you, who will?

❂ **My husband loves me for me! He loves me just the way I am, not for what I look like.** This may be true, but that is no excuse for not taking care of yourself. That sweet man loves you and for that reason alone, you should love yourself enough to be on this earth with him as long as you can. When we allow our health to destroy true love, we hurt the one who loves us the most.

❂ **I have too much weight to lose. It will take too long and I just don't have time.** This is just your perfectionism talking again. Why does there have to be a timetable? Establishing new habits will set you on your journey to a lifetime of good health.

❂ **I really do love my chocolate.** Do you love your chocolate more than you love yourself and life? When we deprive ourselves, it is no wonder we have to eat the whole box to get satisfied. It is not the chocolate we are craving, it is the love that we feel when we eat it.

❂ **I can't eat that weird, awful-tasting diet food!** That is because you have never eaten healthy food. True, food that has become known as "diet food" is tasteless. Taste comes from real food, not from processed clutter.

⊛ **After all, I am healthy: I have good blood pressure and I have no problem with my cholesterol.** There is no doctor in the world who is going to tell you that you are healthy! You are not healthy if you are obese and sedentary.

⊛ **I have been this way a long time and it has not hurt me yet.** No, not yet, sweetie, but obesity is killing a whole generation of us. We are not immune. Wake up and recognize your lies.

⊛ **I am carrying around one hundred extra pounds and that alone makes me strong.** Strong calves, but that is about it. Try walking up a flight of stairs and see if you are out of breath.

⊛ **I don't want to "deny" myself.** Would you rather feed your face than deprive yourself of good, healthy food? The truth is you are denying yourself good health.

I know there are many more where these came from. My dear friend Michele and I came up with this list while driving in the car one day. It was amazing to see our faces as we each came up with yet another one. This was all about getting honest with ourselves and with each other. Saying them out loud was almost scary, too, but when they came out of our mouths, it seemed that the lies we were living just disappeared. Now as I am typing them up I know these lies are going to help others realize how they have been deceiving themselves for many years.

We don't have to betray ourselves with these fabrications. We can accept the fact that Body Clutter is not healthy. Holding on to this kind of clutter is the most unloving thing you can do to yourself. As you release yourself from one lie after another, you will be releasing the Body Clutter with it. Your new attitude is going to change not only the way you think, but your physical body as well. What you think about, you bring about.

## Using Illness as an Excuse

When we live in denial we are unable to eliminate any of our Body Clutter and we come up with excuses. You have heard these excuses come out of your mouth: I've been sick, I have this or that disease, my thyroid won't let me lose weight, my metabolism is messed up. Well, the only true statement is that your metabolism is messed up because you don't eat often enough and move enough.

We put labels on ourselves all the time. Why do we do that? I feel that the use of labels is another form of making an excuse. Those excuses are not for anyone but us. It is to make us feel better because we don't like the Body Clutter we have collected. When are we going to recognize those excuses for what they really are? They are another form of Body Clutter—the kind that is in our head and helps us continue to fool ourselves into believing that it is not our fault that the Body Clutter has collected on our hips and thighs.

Our whole lives, we have been labeled by our families. We grew up hearing that we were lazy and stupid. We were also accused of never being able to finish anything. Now we hear it from ourselves. As a result of hearing those negative words, we have been brainwashed into actually believing them.

Pam Young and Peggy Jones coined the label SHE: Sidetracked Home Executive. It is a cute label and it helps us identify with each other. I guess some labels have a good purpose. But keep in mind that labels can become crutches, too. We use our labels as excuses to whine. Whining is not allowed, not even with the preface that this is not a whine, it is just a fact. To me it is still a whine. I get the same reaction when someone says, "Trust Me!" My first thought is to watch my back.

Now listen very closely. We are not our diseases! I have said this before and I will continue to hammer this home. We may have problems that have names, but they do not have to take over our souls. We have to learn to live with them, but we do not have to become the poster children for them. Having knowledge can help us adapt our lives to deal with problems, but you can't give in to them by taking them on as part of yourself and using them as excuses for collecting Body Clutter.

Here are the facts: We are the ones who put the junk food in our mouth and we are the ones who have a permanent indentation in our favorite chair. This is what has caused our Body Clutter to accumulate slowly, an ounce here and an ounce there. A friend told me the other day that if you gained an ounce every four days, in ten years you would increase your weight by approximately sixty pounds. That is only six pounds a year, but it all adds up.

Someone asked me the other day if I had a goal weight. I

said no because my only goal was to see a slight decrease (as in two-tenths of a pound) every other day or so. The most amazing part of this type of goal is I am enjoying watching the process. I get up and weigh myself and I am not afraid of the number. I am not that number any more than I am the size of my clothes or the color of my hair.

Be who you are, accept yourself, love the inside, and do not look at yourself with disdain. When you stop making excuses you will begin to open up your wings to FLY!

### Body Clutter Mission

Open your friend, the Body Clutter Control Journal. This is a friend that you can be honest with because you are your own best friend. This friend does not criticize your spelling or grammar. Just tell her the truth.

What excuses do you make to yourself for having Body Clutter? Don't hold back! List them all!

# 5. Forgiveness

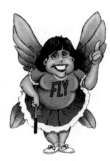

*FlyLady*

In our all-or-nothing, SHE mentality (perfectionism), when we mess up we give up! We have all done it. I have a friend who lost a lot of weight on a no-carb diet. She would stick to it religiously for six months and then out of the blue came cravings and she would eat a candy bar. As a result of her perfectionism, she would see this puny little candy bar as a failure and she would quit following her meal plan, even though she had been so good about following it. Oh, my! Did you hear what I said? When she ate the candy bar, she was not "good" anymore. She did not feel worthy enough to be nice to herself after she had messed up! She needed to be punished, and what better way than to gain her weight back? She was throwing her whole life away over one mistake.

So what do we do when we make a little mistake or even a big one? We are not perfect and we will never be, so the sooner we get rid of our perfectionist thinking when it comes to food, or anything else we do, the faster we are going to be in control of our actions. Right now when we mess up we react like a child who has gone outside the lines on the picture she is coloring. We just want to wad up the paper and throw it away. We can't do that with our body. This is the only body we have.

We have to practice being nice to ourselves. That little candy bar should not be the beginning of a runaway-train eating binge. I think that part of this attitude comes from feeling deprived of the things that we really want, or think we want, when we put ourselves on a diet. When we do eat something we have not had in a long time, we want to continue to indulge ourselves. We have to learn that one bite is enough and does not set us up for failure. Limiting ourselves to only one bite is a celebration when we could have eaten the whole thing. The attitude, "Oh, well, I messed up so I might as well eat a hot fudge sundae and a huge bowl of macaroni and cheese" is self-defeating.

This scenario relates to our lack of forgiveness for our imperfections. Have you ever held a grudge? A grudge is just a bitter pill we take that destroys our soul and doesn't even hurt the person whom we are not forgiving. When are we going to learn that the cure for this bitter disease is that we must first forgive ourselves for our past and quit punishing ourselves for every little mistake?

In our mind, forgiveness is hard to come by, but it is no more difficult than choosing between white or black socks. I know to you this may sound way too simple. We make it difficult because we want the person who has wronged us to make some sort of amends for his or her mistreatment of us. In the same way, we find it hard to forgive ourselves for our mistakes. Why? Are we using those mistakes as just another excuse to abuse ourselves? Is it the foundation for our Body Clutter? Just as we have to love our neighbor in order to love ourselves, we must first forgive ourselves before we can let go of the bitterness we have toward those who have wronged us.

Guilt is the lack of forgiveness manifested in physical anxiety. We have suffered with some form of guilt our whole lives. We don't have to live this way any longer. When you are stuck in the revolving door of guilt and unforgiveness, it is hard to break free. It seems like you are going someplace, but if the truth be known, you are just traveling in a vicious circle that reaps only Body Clutter, with depression, martyrdom, and perfectionism fueling your trapped feelings.

In order to jump clear of those revolving doors you have to forgive yourself for the past. Accept that all the bad things that have ever happened to you were just stepping-stones to a new way of living. Make up your mind to forgive the part you had in those bad choices and press forward in your quest for happiness. You are never going to jump free of that vicious cycle if you are always looking back at the past. You have to let go of those years and accept that you are who you are because of those choices, and thank God for a new way of looking at them. Then release the bad choices and move on. No amount of whining, pining, anger, or self-abuse is going to change what happened in the past. Today is a new day, a new beginning, and a new way of living, free of the guilt because you have made the choice to forgive. I am not saying that you have to forget, but you don't have to constantly dwell on the mistakes of your past. You have learned from them and now you can take a new path without having to turn your back on the present and the future.

Once you have forgiven yourself, you can move on to forgiving others. The most amazing thing happens when you are not burdened by the evil that others do. You are free to FLY! I have had to work very hard on this one. Subconsciously, I was living in rebellion and I didn't even realize it.

Many years ago my ex-husband would look at me in disgust when we went out to dinner, although at the time I probably weighed only 150 pounds. His disdainful look was followed by his taking a roll off my plate. That would make me so angry, but did I ever say anything? No! I just took it! In the back of my mind I decided that no one was going to tell me what I could and could not eat! So I justified eating anything and everything with that attitude. Can I say Body Clutter here? It was probably that attitude that caused my weight gain. I was going to show him! It was a bitter pill that I took to hurt him, but it really didn't faze him in the least. All I did was collect Body Clutter to repel him and it hurt my health. I don't have to live that way any longer.

I have forgiven him for his mistreatment toward me!

He didn't know how to express himself in a loving way. I don't have to make excuses for his behavior. I just had to forgive myself for allowing him to push my buttons, and then I was able to forgive him. With saying these words I have released the rebellion that has controlled my behavior all these years. It feels like a huge weight has been lifted from my shoulders. He is of no consequence to me. I will not allow his inability to love me to hurt me anymore. I now love myself, and there is no greater love.

When we forgive ourselves and others we are loving ourselves first! For many years I have lived with a wonderful man. I have been very happy in our relationship. I always thought that being happy would make the Body Clutter disappear. It wasn't until I released the anger, rebellion, and grudge by forgiving myself and my ex-husband that I started to see a change in my attitude and on my scale!

One of the most potent things in this world is forgiveness. In my estimation, the power to forgive and accept forgiveness is the key to releasing one's internal bondage. Forgiving is empowering—asking yourself for forgiveness as well as extending it to others.

*Leanne*

We lock ourselves into prisons of self-doubt, self-hatred, and loathing. We blame ourselves for a myriad of circumstances in our lives, with a lot of them being stuff that was beyond our control—even the things that were within our control (like choosing a mate, making a decision about accepting a job or going to college, eating food that we know we should avoid, etc.). That we consequently made poor decisions shouldn't be off the forgiveness radar screen. It is when we understand the power to forgive and accept forgiveness (yes, even when it's from ourselves) that we can be released in ways we never imagined or dreamed of.

I've written before about the universal law and principle of sowing and reaping. Forgiveness is a perfect example of this law in action. When the forgiveness is granted (sowing), the benefit (reaping) is immediate and apparent. A burdened-down feeling is replaced by a lightness. There is a feeling of release, a liberation that happens within the soul.

I believe it is at that point that you make room for the good things you want in your life. It's like weeding a garden. If you take out the weeds, you can allow what you want to grow to flourish. And when you take the weeds all the way out—we're talking about grabbing them and pulling them completely out, roots and all—there is room both on the surface and below it. That's an important thing to understand. Forgiveness radiates from the core of your being and will extend itself outward. But it is that inward grace that becomes granted forgiveness, which then becomes transparent in your very countenance. Forgiveness is a supernatural gift that transcends all other creatures, except human beings. Forgiveness is a blessing both to give and to receive. And it is all within your power!

Forgiveness removes the weeds of resentment, anger, and bitterness from your life. I think a lot of us women have a tendency to accidentally water those nasty weeds. We harbor resentments, we feed the anger, and we protect our bitterness. How do we do that? We never forget any details of a hurt and keep them in the forefront of our mind. We talk about the hurt endlessly with our friends. We see therapists to try and deal with it. We take antidepressants and other medications to help take the edge off. We remind ourselves how much that person or event or whatever hurt us, and then we make vows to ourselves that no matter what, we will not allow ourselves ever to be hurt that way again. That kind of thinking only protects a bitter heart but doesn't give us the ground to sow seeds of love. It can't because the forgiveness hasn't happened—yet.

Our heart can be fertile ground for forgiveness once we understand the supernatural power forgiveness has. When we ask for forgiveness, we humble ourselves, admitting things aren't perfect (ah . . . another place where we can release perfectionism!), and we make ourselves vulnerable. It's scary to do this with another human being, but it can be even harder doing it for yourself. We are harder on ourselves than any other human being could ever be. However, understand that the act of forgiveness can truly be the most important way we can love ourselves. Forgiveness, for most of us, needs to be a priority and a starting place in loving ourselves so we can get on with our lives.

The mission for this chapter is on getting the healing you need through forgiveness. It is my heartfelt prayer that you will take this opportunity to allow the unforgiveness in your soul to melt when doing this important exercise. Watch what happens when you do! Your life will begin to fill up with the stuff you do want in it, and I promise this will have an impact on dealing with your Body Clutter as well. Enjoy the journey!

## Body Clutter Mission

This is one of the most cathartic writing assignments you will ever do. Open your Body Clutter Control Journal and share your hurt and anger with your best friend—you!

Do you have someone you are angry with? Write down why you are mad and get it out of you. Write hard and fast! No one else is going to read this.

When you are finished, you can tear it up. We like to call it a brain dump.

Once you get the anger out of you, you can begin the healing process. We are not telling you to forget the hurt, but forgiveness is the key to letting it go. Just grab your pen and don't let your perfectionism stop you in your journey.

# 6. BabySteps

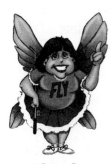

FlyLady

While we all want instant gratification, we must be patient with ourselves. Just as a baby learns to walk little by little, step by step, we apply this principle of gradual change to our Body Clutter. BabySteps are exactly what you think they are. When infants start to move on their own, they begin by scooting along and then crawling. As this becomes more natural, they start to stand and take their first steps; at first they are slow, clumsy, and awkward. These initial steps are a balancing act. They are teetering and cautious, small and short, but as infants adapt to this new skill, they become more and more comfortable with their newfound independence.

These same BabySteps are what we have to allow ourselves to take. So many times in our quest to get thin, get healthy, get whatever it is we are searching for, we want it to be fast and painless. We talk to ourselves all about will-power and how this time we are not going to fail but, sadly, we do fail over and over again. The reason this happens to us goes back to our own desire and need for instant gratification. We want thin thighs, a flat tummy, firm breasts, and whatever else it is that we have told ourselves is wrong with our body—and we want it *now*. The problem with these needs is that we have set the bar of perfection so high that we can't ever meet our own expectations, and once again we fail.

We have to be willing to deal with our perfectionism, lower our expectations, and take small BabySteps toward our ultimate goal: living a longer, healthier, and happier life. Instead of setting ourselves up with a rigorous plan to eat only what a mere child could not survive on and an exercise regimen that even professional athletes couldn't keep up with, we have to take a step back and look at what is realistic.

Realistic can mean that we look at what we are eating and see what small changes we can make that would help our bodies function better and be healthier. If you are drinking five sodas a day, you can take a BabyStep and eliminate just one or two of those. If you are not exercising or moving at all, you could take a BabyStep and add five minutes of movement to your day. If you are beating yourself up every day about how you look and feel, you can take a BabyStep and remind yourself that you are a very special person and deserve to feel good about yourself because you are special just because you are *you*!

Using BabySteps to deal with Body Clutter really comes down to three areas that we have to be willing to take our time and deal with in ways that are doable. They are Food, Attitude, and Movement. Each of these stands alone, but they are also closely woven into the fabric of a healthy life.

## Food

Food is the fuel that allows our body to function, and movement is what burns the fuel. Just like a car, if you put in bad fuel, it will not run well, and if you let a car sit idle for long periods of time, it will run poorly or not at all. When we choose to put food into our body that is not good for us, we become tired, lethargic, and cranky, and we move less. When we sit idle for too long, our lethargy increases and we move even less. See how these two are so closely intertwined?

We start with BabyStepping our eating habits. I have a tendency not to eat breakfast, sometimes skip lunch, and then eat a big dinner. This pattern is not good for me. My Sweet Darling tells me so all the time. I know from Leanne that when I don't eat, my body thinks I don't have enough food and goes into preservation mode and my metabolism slows down. This makes so much sense when you look at it from a starvation/survival physiology. No wonder I have never been able to declutter the extra weight I have been carrying around for years!

So in order to see a change in our Body Clutter, we are going to have to change our eating habits. The amount of food I have been taking in has been just right to keep me from adding more clutter to my body, but it is too much if I want to try to declutter my body just a little. So with tweaking and playing games with my metabolism and reducing my intake just a little, I will be able to see some change in a few months. I am not trying to fit into a bathing suit or anything that extreme. I just want to be healthy and live for a long time. I deserve to feel good in my skin and celebrate my life with my Sweet Darling, not huff and puff when I go up a flight of stairs! Heart disease affects one in three women. It is time we all did something to make ourselves healthier!

**Attitude**

There is something else that adds to the mix and that is our attitude, which is shaped by our emotions. Our emotions can range from happy to sad, from excitement to anger, from joy to tears in 0 to 60 mph in under five seconds flat! We are emotionally affected by food and movement starting from when we talk ourselves into the latest fad diet or exercise craze to the self-defeating feelings we suffer from when we fail. We beat ourselves up over how we can't do anything right, and so the cycle continues. This is where it stops! We have to be willing to stop beating ourselves up and take BabySteps in changing our attitude.

**Movement**

BabySteps will help get us moving. We don't have to be a physical therapist or trainer to know that moving is good for us! Good for our hearts and good for our bodies. We can even play a game with ourselves so that we don't think of this as the e-word!

We can do anything for 15 minutes! That is all we are talking about—getting off our Frannies and moving. It can be walking, dancing, aerobics, or anything else that you think is fun. Some of you may even include your furry friends for some movement. If you don't love it, you won't do it. Use BabySteps to find a way of moving that you enjoy. Move to the beat of your own drum. Some of us need variety, while others love doing the same thing each day. It does not matter what you do, just as long as you are up and moving—and having fun!

Our BabySteps for movement are to move a little in the morning and a little more in the evening. I want to increase my metabolism so that I can reduce some of the clutter on my body. Since I have been walking on my treadmill three to five times a week, I have not noticed a difference in my clothes. This tells me that the walking has been helpful at keeping my body just the way it is. In order to declutter just a little each week, I am going to have to do a little more. If I jump in and force myself to do a full hour on the treadmill, I will only make myself dread getting on it, and the treadmill will become a dreadmill and I won't do it. I know me better than anyone else. Why do you think I started by shining my sink? That was all I had to do. I did not burden or punish myself by trying to do too much too fast. I took a BabyStep and the result has been peace in my home. *Nothing else* had ever worked before! This time it worked because I took care of my needs by BabyStepping while establishing new habits.

I want moving always to be part of my daily routine and I don't want to hate doing it. I want it to be as natural to me as my habits of getting up and getting dressed to shoes and shining my sink are for me now.

Because I have begun to BabyStep with some movement and I have been getting on my treadmill first thing in the morning, I have had to adapt my routine just a little. Here is what happened yesterday: I got up, hit the shower as usual, and then did the rest of my simple Morning Routine. After that I hopped on the treadmill and started to glisten (in the South, women don't sweat). When I finished I really needed another shower! So this morning I am going to do my moving first thing and then start my day over with a shower, at which point I may even pretend I am getting up for the first time this morning!

Our routines are not supposed to be straitjackets. They should be adaptable in order to fit our lifestyle. Here is the hard part for me: I have to make a new rule for myself—I can't sit down in my chair and go to work being FlyLady until I have started my day over with exercise and a shower! I will practice this for a few days until it begins to feel comfortable.

It does not matter if you start BabyStepping with two minutes or fifty! All I care about is that each day you get up and do just a little more than the day before. It feels so good to take those first steps toward Blessing Your Heart. We can do this, and we are not going to crash and burn— we are going to build new heart-healthy habits that are going to stay with us for life!

Are you taking care of yourself? You know what I am talking about: drinking enough water, wearing decent shoes, and pacing yourself. Have you talked to your doctor recently? If your shins start hurting, then you need to walk on a softer surface or get better athletic shoes. Shin splints are painful and will keep you from moving. Do not suffer in silence. I have found if I walk for exercise on concrete or pavement, even with the best shoes, my shins hurt. So I choose to walk on a treadmill or in the woods.

You have to take care of yourself when you move. That means protecting your little tootsies, too! In one accident, the mover wasn't wearing athletic shoes and while trying to keep up with his dear wife, he stubbed his little toe! He had to wear open-toed shoes to work the next day. Poor little pinky toe! Shoes protect our feet and energize our steps. Wear them! I have one friend who broke her foot running barefoot on the beach because she didn't want to get sand in her shoes! What is a little sand compared to a broken bone? You are worth taking care of. No one else can do this for you. Please, really give your heart a little workout. You can have fun with this!

On the news recently I saw a couple of ships returning to port after being out to sea for over nine months. One sailor was searching for his wife. When he finally found her, he could not believe the transformation she had undergone. She had decluttered her body! So think of it this way: I have told you many times that decluttering your home is like giving birth to a new you—it takes about nine months to establish your routines so that the habits evolve and become part of you. Let's do the same with our personal transformation. We can do this—one BabyStep at a time!

I have been FLYing for a long time! This love has kept me from setting myself up for failure many times. I celebrate my small successes and don't beat myself up because I didn't do more! As with your routines, the more you practice, the easier it gets! Let's BabyStep to a new way of thinking.

Leanne

What attracted me to FlyLady's system was the no-guilt aspect of getting my house in order. I could do as much or as little as I wanted as long as I did *something* (like get dressed to shoes or shine my sink). Doing something, even a little something, would help me progress and new habits would be formed. And that's what we have to address—just doing something: making progress in feeding ourselves well, moving a little more each day, and keeping our minds and attitudes focused.

When FlyLady and I were working on this book, she told me how much she wanted to make sure that you love your body just as it is and that you know you are all beautiful. FLYing is all about loving yourself and taking care of yourself. The habit of exercise is one way you can do that and

FlyLady's doing it! Her treadmill probably has logged enough miles to get her to Toledo and back by now! But she started BabyStepping on that treadmill! You can do the same with nutrition. Start with adding one salad a week with a meal. See what you've done? You've BabyStepped up your nutrition a notch. Make the salad a habit and then start looking at some other things you can do—when you're ready. Like maybe a piece of fruit instead of doughnuts or rich pastries, water instead of soda, or how about adding broccoli to your shopping list this week?

When you drink your water, when you exercise, and when you feed yourself and your family good stuff, you feel better! You look better too—clear skin and eyes, extra energy, and a little spring in your step.

## BabySteps Keep You Balanced

My mom and dad went to Europe when I was a senior in high school. They started in Los Angeles and stopped in New York, then finally landed in London. Part of the itinerary for the trip involved a quick jaunt to Paris. My mom had never been there and was looking forward to the adventure. During the quick trip to Paris, one of the plane's engines malfunctioned and they were forced to make an emergency landing. The captain explained that they wouldn't crash, but that it would be necessary to land prematurely because the plane wasn't balanced.

This is what happens to us when we're out of whack— the balance is off and so are we. Hormones are screaming, and we're constantly fighting fatigue and a whole host of other related complaints. We need balance desperately, but how do we attain it?

Let's go back to the airplane for a minute. The plane is our body and those two engines represent our metabolism. We need both of those engines to keep our body balanced. Keeping our metabolism fired up requires movement and fuel, and that's what we're talking about right now, but in a language we can understand—BabySteps. Our old perfectionist habits want to rear their ugly heads and tell us to do this in a way that will not only guarantee burning out but will also cause us to give up and never want to tackle our Body Clutter issues again.

If we look realistically at our body, we will see excess baggage and a lack of fitness. These two traits feed off each other. The less we move, the more baggage goes onto our body. The more we consume, the less energy we have to move because we are weighted down. This produces bad feelings that make us want to eat more and move even less. We have to put an end to this downward spiral and stop ourselves from crashing before we ever get off the ground.

It is time to use our BabySteps to start our journey. Imagine that you have to ascend several steps before you are ready to begin. Each one of these steps is a new way of thinking or a new habit that is going to help us on our adventure.

## Body Clutter Mission

Use your Body Clutter Control Journal to help you build your routine one BabyStep at a time. This Body Clutter Mission is to get you thinking about small, doable steps in all three areas of Food, Movement, and Attitude. Do not let your perfectionism make this simple task into a mission impossible.

Be sure that the BabySteps you implement today will not cause you to feel overwhelmed when it comes to your already established routines. Do not pile on too much too fast or you will crash and burn.

List one BabyStep that will help you be more aware of what food you are putting in your mouth.

When it comes to movement, what is a simple BabyStep that is doable for you today?

List one BabyStep that will help you with your perfectionist attitude.

# 7. Building Your Routines

The joy of routines cannot be overstated. As with anything in life that is worth doing, there is a certain amount of effort required on a regular basis to make it to that goal. We call them "routines" here because that effort is scheduled daily. You take the Baby-Steps and add them together to create a customized routine developed by you for what you need. It's amazing what routines can accomplish in all areas of life, including the area of Body Clutter.

*Leanne*

When we bless our homes by keeping them neat and in order, we BabyStep through our routines. My morning routine includes making my bed, collecting the dirty clothes, throwing a load in the wash, and wiping down the bathrooms. I also make sure my children are on task to get their routines accomplished as well. When I do these things, everything runs well. When I don't, the smoothness of the day is lost and I inevitably lose momentum.

How true this is for eating and moving as well! In order to incorporate healthy eating into your life, it needs to be a part of your routines. The BabySteps include keeping a grocery list, doing the shopping, and making sure you are prepared. You also have to figure out how you need to eat, when you need to eat, and what would be the best fuel possible to keep you FLYing and happy. When these BabySteps are incorporated into a routine, big things happen: You have a greater inner resolve to go forward, you can see your way to a new goal or two, and you start to feel almost invincible. It's true! That's how empowering having routines is. And the very coolest part of including food in your routine is that the Body Clutter will fall off with less effort than you think. This will seriously astound you with how simple the whole thing really is.

Just like BabySteps make up routines, eating several small meals stokes up our metabolism. Both FlyLady and I do this, and we're both so excited at the changes we are starting to see. Neither of us feels deprived, neither of us is ever hungry and, most important, the urge to pig out due to low blood sugar has been quelled! That is a major breakthrough for both of us. You don't have to do things our way—we're just sharing with you what works for us. While we both eat five or six small meals every day, we do it very differently from each other—there are no perfect routines for everyone, just routines that work well for each of us.

Using each meal of the day and snacks as BabySteps to build your routines will help you keep your metabolism stoked and your fuel burning. Here's what eating five or six meals a day looks like: breakfast, lunch, and dinner, plus two to three snacks. For a snack between meals, FlyLady eats eleven almonds; I eat a piece of string cheese and an apple—I will occasionally eat almonds, but I have a tendency to eat more than just eleven. This is called knowing yourself and knowing your limits—all important, necessary components to getting this FLYing thing down when you're trying to lose the Body Clutter. You have to be willing not to get bogged down by the simplicity. We have ourselves convinced from previous failures that there is no way that something simple can work for us. It has to be difficult and complex to work, right? No pain, no gain, right? Wrong!

The first time I had the opportunity to work with a personal trainer, he said something that stuck with me. I had heard it before, but this time I *listened*. He said that in order to make lasting change, you need to burn more than you take in. It's that simple! Once again there's that simplicity thing. We think of exercising as something that takes up so much time that we just can't find a place for it in our busy lives, or we go into overkill and push ourselves so far so fast that we inevitably burn out and quit . . . again! We have to believe that we can take small BabySteps that are simple to put together into small routines. We can add a morning walk to our day, not a forty-five-mile hike in the woods or a twenty-five-mile jogging marathon. Try an after-dinner walk. Start with small movements that eventually will evolve into a medley of move-ment—routines.

Another thing that often stands in the way of reaching one's goals is procrastination. If you put off planning, you won't have anything to work with. In desperation you will be grabbing all the wrong things to eat and then turn around and feel guilty and angry that you don't have what you need, can't make it happen, and then just give up, de-feated. Understand that the saboteur is procrastination and the lack of planning—and nothing else!

We all are living busy lives. We have families, careers, and a whole host of commitments. But just remember this: Your priorities will dictate your plan. Procrastination is the polar opposite to that statement and will pull you down faster than anything else. Don't succumb to this evil siren's call. Stand your ground, make your plan, and go forward. BabySteps and routines will add balance to your busy life. You can do this!

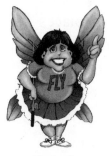

*FlyLady*

### The Dance of Routines

Have you ever tried to learn a new dance step or an aerobic workout? Not me. I have two left feet and I once won an award for being the most-improved, aerobically challenged person in our class. The same goes for learning a golf swing or how to cast a fly-fishing rod. The first time you do it, things just don't feel right. The muscles in your arms and legs just don't go where you think they should. The problem isn't with the muscles in your arms and legs; it is with the muscle that is between your ears. This goes back to wanting things *now* and not wanting to slow down and learn the individual steps that it takes to be able to do the dance. We want to watch and, presto, be able to do it ourselves.

Your brain is what works those muscles. If you have not gotten the movement choreographed in your head, your limbs will not follow because you have not given them the directions. Routines are just BabySteps put together into a dance that makes your day FLY!

One time I learned a fly-fishing casting technique in the rain, riding in a car. In my mind I put every movement into place over and over again. I got out of the car and performed it without a flaw. I had mentally practiced it in the car, I had developed the right rhythm, and the rest of it flowed into place.

You have to be willing to take very small BabySteps toward building routines for food, movement, and attitude. We don't expect you to try to do a full-blown routine to start with. We know that you will be tempted to create a long and torturous routine at first because it goes back to our all-or-nothing thinking. You have to be willing to step out in faith and trust that the small BabySteps you put together with other small BabySteps will create a realistic and doable routine. Putting together your small routines will reinforce your rhythm and your dance will glide you through your daily rounds. Here are examples of putting BabySteps together for a routine:

☻ You never eat breakfast or you eat an unhealthy breakfast. The BabyStep is not a full-out breakfast buffet, but a piece of fruit and a whole-grain muffin or cereal. The BabyStep is making this small but healthy change.

☻ You sleep as late as you possibly can and then rush out the door to sit in the car or at a desk. The BabyStep is not getting up three hours early and doing a workout that is so physically strenuous that you need to go back to bed to recover. Instead it is getting up twenty minutes earlier than usual and taking a small 15-minute walk in your neighborhood. The BabyStep is adding a little more movement to your day than yesterday.

☻ Your evening meals are usually ordered through a squawk box at a drive-thru window. The BabyStep is not having dinner brought to you by the pizza delivery guy. Instead, dinner is planned ahead of time with a menu and grocery list. The BabyStep is having a small, doable plan instead of grinding your teeth in stress over what to feed the family or giving in to the quick, unhealthy fix.

☻ You have decided that getting thin or healthy is just too hard and have given up completely. The BabyStep is not beating yourself up over and over, thinking that you are a failure, but to take a deep breath and remind yourself that you are worth taking care of. The BabyStep is slowly learning to let go of the Stinking Thinking of the past.

☻ A BabyStep is choosing one new thing to become a habit.

A routine is adding those habitual BabySteps together. Do you see how adding new steps as the first ones become automatic will help your rhythm? Once you have achieved making one BabyStep a habit you will have confidence in the part you know, and adding a new portion does not seem so difficult.

✿ That is exactly how I established my routines—one habit at a time, from shining my sink to getting dressed to shoes every day. I have now added BabySteps for eating and moving to create routines for my Body Clutter. You can do this, too. I don't want you to stumble and fall because you don't have the dance steps down pat. Practice them! Having your steps written out on paper will help you more than anything. Decide which steps are your lead steps. BabySteps are the key.

✿ We have tried the all-or-nothing system and it does not work for most of us. We do too much too fast in order to see immediate results and then we crash and burn, and we have failed again. I don't want you to fail. I want for you what I have—peace, and this peace came by practicing the steps to my routine. Now I glide through my day and the rhythm of my routines keeps me dancing to my FLYing music.

✿ As we move forward into dealing with our Body Clutter, we are going to address more deeply the three key factors for which we have to be able to establish BabySteps and routines: food, movement, and attitude. We will take them one BabyStep at a time and show you how to make good healthy choices for a longer and healthier life.

## Body Clutter Mission

Your Body Clutter Control Journal is where you are going to write down your routines. This does not have to be perfect. You are on your way!

A routine is a series of habits done in a specific order, much like a dance step. Use the habits you already have to help you incorporate new habits. When you partner an established habit with a new habit, you are now practicing new routines that will help you on your Body Clutter journey.

What habits have you already established in a normal morning and evening routine? Write them down. Now add a new, small BabyStep connected to it for you to practice.

Do you have a calendar and stickers that you can use to chart your success? As you practice a new habit, celebrate your accomplished ones by giving yourself a star, a happy face, or any other symbol of your success.

# 8. Food

The supersize mentality is a type of behavior modification in its most negative form. The media figures into the equation by helping form our decisions through repetitive indoctrination. Supersizing it has replaced old-fashioned gluttony pushed on us by all forms of media: print, radio, movies, and TV.

*Leanne*

What do you see in your mind's eye when you hear the words "fast food"? Do you see golden arches and a clown named Ronald? Or is it more like a bearded Southern gentleman whispering promises of perfectly fried chicken?

I believe drive-thru places prey on women who are living chaotic lives. They know our profiles and they've set convenient traps for us throughout our cities. They know we will show up—and we do—because it's so easy. We bargain with ourselves as we supersize it and promise to make a really healthy meal tomorrow, but tomorrow's healthy meal never comes because we haven't planned for it. Our just-this-one-time-won't-hurt rationalization turns into a lifestyle.

I don't need to tell you that eating the bulk of your food from a drive-thru burger joint is bad for you. You already know that. With a little sustained effort (BabySteps), you can completely transform your nutritional profile and improve your health and that of your family's dramatically.

I know there are times when it's easy just to drive through those beckoning arches and throw burgers to the kids in the backseat and finish your drive home from soccer. I most definitely understand the whole concept of busy. Been there, done that, got the T-shirt. I also know how tempting it is to be sucked in by the frozen-food trap, especially the "lite" stuff. But read the label and ask yourself: do you know what half those words mean? Can you pronounce them? Do you know what they do? Do you really want them taking up residence in your body?

Just because you're busy doesn't mean you can't build good food into your routine and make good nutrition a part of your life. The amazing thing is that doing this will help your Body Clutter dissipate naturally with time. The secret of the whole thing is being selective and careful. You deserve the best—don't throw junk into your body merely to fill the void.

## Feeding Souls

Think of food in different terms: In the long run, the easy way is really the hard way because nutritionally you end up short-changing yourself and your family and setting yourselves up for health problems that will appear later. When you miss the boat on feeding yourself and your family well, there are extreme consequences: Body Clutter starting at an early age for your children, degenerating health for you, and just plain feeling rotten. One of the key reasons we feel physically run down, moody, and not wanting to do much of anything is often improper nutrition. We feel crummy because we haven't given our body what it needs.

It's so easy to forget that a part of our job raising a family is to teach them to be nutritionally responsible and that it all begins with a good example. It helps to remember that we need to face the feeding of a family and the feeding of ourselves with a certain amount of seriousness. After all, we are feeding souls, not filling holes. That includes you, too. Don't forget!

All it takes is 15 minutes a day to improve just a little bit. Sit down with your grocery list and make *sure* you've got some healthy stuff included. You don't need to have an all-or-nothing attitude about this—I'm not suggesting only tofu and collard greens for the rest of your life, or even to completely ban fast food. Just balance the fast-food option against the fact that your body will feel better if you feed it better. We just need to combine common sense with a tiny bit of planning—a BabyStep.

Here's a very simple BabyStep to start: Include a salad, or an additional salad, as part of this week's meals. Someone told me that making sure there was something fresh and green in her grocery cart for the week was a lightbulb moment for her because it was easy to remember. Something fresh and green from the produce section was like color-coding her shopping cart to take better care of her family.

You can, too!

### Take Heart—The Big Picture

Women are four to six times more likely to die of heart problems than breast cancer. If one of your health goals is to keep your heart as healthy as possible (good move, too—kind of critical in the staying alive scheme of things), then, once again, you need to step up to the plate nutritionally—breakfast, lunch, and dinner plate, that is. There's more to food than just trying to satisfy your appetite.

Knowing what nutrients your heart needs to operate optimally will not only do it good but will keep the rest of you healthy as well. There are foods that give the heart a nutritional advantage and provide protection in the form of antioxidants. Free radicals break down our health and naturally occur in the processing and digesting of food. However, there are certain foods that are rich in antioxidants and will promote good health. To understand free radicals, think about what happens to a bike left out in the elements—it rusts. Putting your bike in the garage will help prevent that from occurring. Eating foods rich in antioxidants is like providing a nutritional garage for your heart.

### Vitamins—Mother Nature's Way

Foods rich in vitamins A, C, and E (the antioxidants you need), with all their natural corresponding phytochemicals, are, front and center, the best choices for heart health.

Foods abundant in vitamin A include eggs, dark-green leafy vegetables, broccoli, and yellow and orange veggies.

Vitamin C is associated with citrus fruits but is also present in large amounts in bell peppers (especially red ones), broccoli, strawberries, and kiwis.

Vitamin E is present in leafy greens, avocados, whole grains, and nuts and seeds.

You don't need to memorize these, just know that when you BabyStep with your grocery cart by adding fresh fruits and colorful vegetables you are adding heart-healthy habits to your life. These same nutrients will help keep you healthy for other health issues that may concern you, like cancer and other diseases. So take heart! Keeping your heart healthy is something you can do by eating a wide variety of healthy foods like some of the ones mentioned above.

## Portion Control

This was the big lesson for me—less is more. Just because it's healthy doesn't mean we need to strap on the bottomless feedbag. While quality is very important, so is the quantity. Healthy food doesn't give you license to pig out. FlyLady said earlier that she even pigged out on rice cakes. So it's back to square one with an old-fashioned value: portion control.

We buy into the notion that the "perfect" diet or exercise machine will do it for us. We buy the food, the equipment, the supplements, the memberships—the whole nine yards, throwing hundreds of dollars into our quest to rid ourselves of Body Clutter. It's not our fault; the diet industry has packaged it that way—that's how it's sold and we've fallen for it more than once. But here's the kicker: We ourselves hold the answer, not those diets! We can BabyStep our way into diet freedom and never buy or look at another diet book again, once we understand and come to peace with portion control.

Let's translate that to our plates. What makes up a portion? Well, a portion of protein is 4 to 6 ounces, depending on whom you ask. That's roughly the size and height of a deck of cards. A good point of reference, and one that is always with you, is to measure the portion against the palm of your hand (minus fingers) which is approximately 4 to 6 ounces (unless you have tiny or enormous hands!).

A 1-cup portion is roughly the size of a clenched fist. Likewise, the size of an average potato is that same clenched-fist size. The same with an apple, an orange, or a bunch of grapes. See how easy that is?

It was amazing how much I was overeating! Although I was eating healthfully, I wasn't losing any Body Clutter. Portion control is the wake-up call I needed. I've been practicing it and already my stomach feels flatter and my underwear isn't as tight. I judge how I'm doing by my underwear. If I find myself living in Wedgie Land, then I know I have slacked off on watching my portions.

The purpose of portion control is to give you back control of your body, your stomach, and your appetite. You deserve to dictate what you are going to do and how you are going to take care of yourself. Have you ever thought of it this way: A bag of chocolate candies (or whatever food you overly indulge in) is running your life? Think about it. When you eat compulsively, you have given your power away to something that isn't even alive and can't even hold a conversation. We need to get a grip and determine who or what is in charge. If it is you, tell the chocolate candies to shove off and you take the helm. This is your boat—steer it.

That brings me to another thing that just drives me nuts, and that is, do we eat problem foods in moderation or do we abstain? Chocolate (as in chocolate candy, not chocolate cake, etc.) is a problem for me. I can't eat it in moderation. I need to relinquish this food because it is something that damages me. It's just that simple: I can and will live without it. It's not a survival issue. Do I like it? Sure! But I bet if you asked an alcoholic if he liked vodka martinis he'd let you know he thought they were pretty great. They not only didn't do him any favors but were also ruining his body. There are certain people (me included) who need to abstain from certain foods. That particular food has too much power and we need to stay away, plain and simple. But this is a very individual call— some people don't need to be so drastic, others do. It's up to you to call a spade a spade. If it is a problem, make a decision. If you can do moderation, then make a plan and determine just what that looks like. If you can't, perhaps you have to give it up and leave it at the supermarket.

Those who plan for future problems will be more likely to stave them off.

## Burn, Baby, Burn: How to Rev Your Own Engine and Burn More Body Clutter

It's all about metabolism: having an optimally running metabolism vs. a sluggish metabolism. The idea that we're "stuck" and can't lose the Body Clutter is nonsense. I don't buy it and you shouldn't either. The trick is just that—playing tricks on your body and showing it who's boss!

One of the most effective ways I have found to regulate my metabolism is to eat several small meals a day instead of three big ones, or worse, skipping breakfast, grazing for lunch, and pigging out at dinnertime—my old stand-by habit.

Having several small meals a day (I do five—some people even do six) keeps blood sugar levels from wildly fluctuating and keeps me from suddenly bottoming out. When my blood sugar crashes, I want to consume mass quantities of anything I can quickly get in my mouth. That's the pits (in more ways than one) and shoots healthy eating habits in the foot every time.

We're not talking about chowing down on ranch-hand-sized meals here. It's all about stoking the fire of your metabolism a little bit to get it started. For me that means having a very small bowl of bran cereal in the morning. And we're talking *small*. I follow the suggestion on the box of cereal—only 2/3 of a cup. But with that cereal I've just given my body one-third of the fiber I will need for the day, I've put a little something in my tank to get my engine warmed up, and later, when I get hungry, I can eat again.

Let me show you how I am doing it—it's really easy and keeps me from gathering too much clutter. Know what I mean?

**Breakfast**: A couple of eggs with whole-grain toast and a teeny bit of butter on that toast (use whipped, it spreads easily so you use less). Or I will eat cereal as explained above.

**Midmorning Snack**: Low-fat yogurt mixed with low-fat cottage cheese. (The extra protein holds me.)

**Lunch**: Canned tuna, a big green salad with olive oil and rice vinegar, baby carrots, and an apple.

**Afternoon Snack**: Protein drink or bar (high protein/low carb).

**Dinner**: A portion of protein cooked in a low-fat manner (broiled, grilled, poached, etc.), baked squash (or some other yellow or orange veggie), steamed broccoli, and brown rice (if at all—there are already plenty of carbs in the squash).

**Evening Snack**: Low-fat yogurt. Make sure you eat this snack three hours before you go to bed. You don't want to be rolling around on it all night!

Eating many little meals is an effective way to stoke the fire of your metabolism, which is a big key for many people trying to lose their Body Clutter. By eating good stuff more often, you will feel better and won't hit that afternoon low like you used to (you know, when you want to have a nap at 2 o'clock in the afternoon). That is because your blood sugar level won't dip like it does when you're eating three squares a day. This is an ideal way to even out your temperament, too—who knew?

Eating minimeals more often during the day is a great BabyStep because it's not hard to accomplish. It takes a little rearranging of old habits and some forward thinking and planning, but anything of value requires effort, right?

FlyLady always says, "Your house did not get dirty overnight and it's not going to get clean in a day." The same concept plays out when you're dealing with your Body Clutter: You didn't suddenly sprout those thighs overnight—you've been growing them for years. To "ungrow" them, it's going to take a focused effort, just like getting your house in order.

We can do this. BabySteps are our best friend. *No* diet is really going to "work." Maybe it will for a while, but at some point you'll go back to eating the "normal way" and all that extreme effort and deprivation will have added up to a big zero! There is no magic pill, no new magic diet, or movie star exercise video that will suddenly bless you with the body you want with no work. Not gonna happen.

However, I promise you this: If you make the effort,

take your BabySteps, and stay focused on your goals, you will begin to lose your Body Clutter and it will last—for real this time!

### Breakfast Is Your Shiny Sink

When we begin to follow FlyLady's BabySteps in getting our houses in order, our first BabyStep is to shine our sinks. That clean and shining sink represents a new way to do things and becomes a centerpiece to our routines. That sink also offers a renewed sense of hope. Taking BabySteps means going forward, falling down, and jumping back in where you are. We know when we fall back on our old ways that we aren't doomed. All we have to do is go shine our sinks.

When we are trying to deal with Body Clutter, we need to think in terms of our body's "shining sink." For us that is breakfast—giving our body its first fuel up. Everyone has heard that breakfast is the most important meal of the day, but sometimes we just don't feel much like eating first thing in the morning. Eating breakfast, however, is a critical BabyStep toward firing up the metabolism and getting the fat-burning machine working.

This is an important time—it is when you break your fast from not eating all night. It's your body's wake-up call to start operating again full throttle. The message is: Rest is over; it's time to go to work. At this point, your blood sugar is low—you need fuel to get that engine working again.

Starting the day fuelless is like taking a car on a long

journey hoping the reserve tank will get you there and back. I promise you, it's not going to happen. Most likely you will end up eating something greasy from a drive-thru or a bag of something high in fats and carbs because your blood sugar has crashed, or you'll wait till lunch and then eat out of control because you're starving. Let's not even talk about our foul moods due to our blood sugar being in the can. This is not how we're meant to operate and, most important, we deserve better.

The wonderful thing about breakfast is that it's a cheap and easy meal. I'm not talking about the artificially colored, sugary breakfast cereals. That stuff is an overpriced, over-marketed, unhealthy nightmare that doesn't have you or your family's nutritional needs in mind at all.

Many parents tell me that their kids want only the sugary stuff. Let me say this as emphatically as possible: YOU are the parent and YOU can control what goes in your child's cereal bowl every day. Don't give your power to the Madison Avenue marketers.

First thing in the morning it's important to get complex carbs and not simple carbs (whole grains as opposed to white flour) plus a serving of protein. A good example is two eggs and a piece of whole wheat toast, or a breakfast burrito (whole wheat tortilla, a couple of scrambled eggs, and salsa), or a protein smoothie and, if you're on the go, a protein bar and an apple. There are a number of ways to accomplish a healthy start to your day, and I guarantee you will feel better if you "shine your sink" first thing in the morning and get yourself a little healthy breakfast before starting your day.

Here is a list of assorted tips you may find helpful:

☢ *My favorite is the liquid-calorie tip. We've said that you can save yourself over thirty pounds a year if you just give up your soda-a-day habit. But a magazine I was reading recently said that if you gave up two sodas a day and your glass of juice (the whole fresh fruit is better for you anyway), you would lose forty-four pounds in one year. That's the kind of BabyStep I like! Obviously, if you replace the juice and sodas with lemon meringue pie and Snickers bars, the deal is off.*

☢ *Here's a great shape-up tip that I read on the internet. Exercise during TV commercials. Get down on the floor and do a few sit-ups or some push-ups or dance in place for the duration of the commercial break. It's amazing what you can accomplish with BabySteps!*

☢ *If your habit is to mindlessly graze on chips and pretzels and the like, replace them with some dill pickles. You'll get the crunch and the salt without having to deal with the clutter that comes from overeating the other stuff. As a matter of fact, if you eat thirty-two pickles in one sitting, you'll ingest only 160 calories (not that anyone would want to eat thirty-two pickles at one time, but you get what I mean).*

✪ *If you do want to eat chips or pretzels or something else like that, understand that they don't have to be completely off-limits. But be aware of portion control and set some rules for yourself. Don't allow yourself to eat out of a big bag of anything anymore. Somehow we all have the notion that a little bit of grazing doesn't count—until it shows up on our backside and makes our pants hard to put on. Put your chips into a small, zip-topped bag—a serving size (1 ounce)—and be content with that. Otherwise, just buy individual servings that you'd throw in the kids' lunches. They may cost more, but at least you won't be paying for it personally—you know what I mean.*

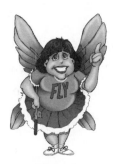

FlyLady

What value do we put on ourselves or our families? Are we willing to ruin our children's relationship with food in order to live up to the values we have had imposed on us by our parents and by the advertising world?

What have those values done to us? I received a letter from Chris (the wife of our web editor Lee) about something she had witnessed at a popular fast-food restaurant. I was just as saddened by this story as she was. I shared this letter with the members of the FlyLady mentoring list and received hundreds of replies that proved to me that we all have been overwhelmed by the result of years of this kind of Stinking Thinking—or shall I call it for what it really is: BODY CLUTTER! Here is the message from Chris:

Dear Marla,

Catie and I went to Wal-mart yesterday, and we stopped off at McDonald's for an ice cream cone. As we were eating our ice cream cone, a mom comes in with her three children. One of the younger children had said she wanted a plain cheeseburger. The mom had then asked her if she wanted a plain cheeseburger or a double cheese-burger. Now keep in mind this little one must have been four years old; so the little one says that she just wants the regular one.

Then the other kids said the same thing (approximate ages for the three girls: ten, seven, and four). The mom tells them that the regular cheeseburger is almost as much as the double burger (the regular is a few cents cheaper than a double). The kids insist they want only a regular but the mom proceeds to buy double cheeseburg-ers for everyone. At this time I am asking myself, Why is she pushing all this extra food on her little kids? Yes, you get more food for your money and I am all for getting the best deal, but a double cheeseburger for a four-year-old?

Anyway, I tell myself maybe she is going to save part of it for later (after all, there has to be an explanation for this). Much to my dismay, she then proceeds to get upset with the little sweetie when she says she is full and doesn't want any more. She tells her that she has just wasted good money and she will not be getting an ice cream with the rest of her sisters. She started to cry and said, "Okay, Mommy, I will finish it." I just couldn't believe it! I felt like pulling that little girl aside and giving her a big hug! My heart was just crying with her.

I just had to tell someone who would get my frustration and heartache over this.

Talk to you later,
Chris

When I read this message I cried as if someone had died. My son called and I could not even talk for a minute; finally I got out that no one had died. Then I read him the message. Now as I am trying to put my feelings down, I think someone did die that moment in McDonald's. It was that little child. She was listening to her God-given instinct to judge when she is full and her mother made her disregard the message that her body was telling her.

All of us have had our little child hurt by this attitude. Just think back to your childhood. Some of us were forced to eat things that made us gag. Others were left at the table for hours until we ate what was on our plates. God help us if we were taken out to eat at a restaurant; the ordeal became so painful that we learned to excuse ourselves to the bathroom so we would not be yelled out for not eating all the food that was on our plate. If we didn't eat it we were wasting good money. What if we were receiving mixed messages from our parents, one parent telling you that you were too fat and the other fussing because you didn't clean your plate? No wonder we don't know how to eat and listen to our bodies. We have had to listen to these generations of brainwashing that taught us that there is value in eating as much as you can because you had paid good money for it.

The idea that we are entitled to as much as we can get has to be stopped. Have you ever noticed how people act at a buffet? They fill up their plates as high as they can. It doesn't matter that they can go back as often as they want. What is this all about? It is about getting all they can for their money. When is enough enough?

Isn't this the same feeling that causes us to fill our homes with clutter? We don't recognize when we are full or even when our homes are full. Now let's take a look at our schedules—we don't even notice that we keep adding more to our calendars. All we do is run, run, run and eat as fast and as much as we can.

In one message we received, a mother said that her mother-in-law had told her children that they were going to hell if they didn't clean their plates! How can anyone come up with something as off-the-wall as that? The last time I checked, gluttony was one of the seven deadly sins. The dictionary defines gluttony as the habit of overeating. We have been doing that for years. It is an ineffective habit that has caused the Body Clutter to creep up on us one meal at a time. All because we were forced to kill off the food-moderating instinct that God gave us in order to appease someone who was bigger than we were and had more power.

We have all been conditioned by a Depression era mentality: We might starve someday; we have to save it for later; get as much as you can before someone else gets it;

waste not, want not; a penny saved is a penny earned; there are starving children in Africa; you have to be saving all the time; use it up, wear it out, make it do, or do without! Some of these adages help us be wise with our money, but when we use them to condition our children to fill their tummies to the point of being sick, then we have taken something good and turned it into evil that will destroy our minds and bodies.

The next time you see a value menu at a fast-food restaurant, ask yourself, "What value is it if you don't need it?" It is not a bargain if you eat more than your body needs. When you do that, you only end up spending more money on medical problems related to obesity and eating disorders.

Life is about choices. When you decided to buy this book, you made a choice. When you decided to read it, you made another choice. Everything you do requires choices. This is what Body Clutter is all about—recognizing that you do have a choice and making the BabyStep choices to change your attitude and your way of living.

Many years ago in a college writing class, I had an assignment to take a walk through the grocery store. We were instructed to describe the market in full detail. Every major grocery store is laid out to entice you to purchase the products. There is always music playing on the intercom system, the lighting is pleasing to the eye, and there are beautiful colors tickling your senses. Not only are they planned to persuade you to purchase, but they lure our children in, too. Take notice of the cereal aisle next time you stroll through it. All the kiddie cereals are on the bottom shelf.

Grocery shopping for me used to be quite simple. I would buy the same old things because I don't like change. Maybe it wasn't because I don't like change as much as it was that I don't like to make choices. I didn't even realize that there were choices other than brand affiliation. I guess I thought food was food and just because I bought it and ate it, that it was good enough.

Leanne has taught me so much about nutritional choices. In my quest for a healthier lifestyle, I have come to realize that some food choices can be negative nutrition. Imagine eating something that robs you of the nutrients you already have in your body. My new way of living has given me a renewed respect for every morsel that I put into my body. I actually think before I purchase, prepare, and consume anything.

## Looking at Labels

Now my trip to the grocery store has become a game for me. I am no longer roaming every aisle looking for inspiration for what to cook; I go shopping with a purpose. I have my list. Instead of traipsing up and down each aisle looking for what I used to buy on a regular basis—you know, the same old stuff—I now look at the labels.

Me, looking at the nutrition labels! Until recently I would never have considered doing that. This has been quite an educational feat for me. The first time I did it, I had Kelly by my side and Leanne on the phone. They were trying to teach me to make good choices on my own. Leanne and Kelly have been doing this for years. Leanne taught Kelly how to help me make choices when it came to reducing my carbohydrate intake for my diabetes. They were my guides until I understood on my own.

I learned that carbs come in the form of sugars and starches. When you see that number on a label you also have to look for the amount of fiber that is in the food. If an apple has 24 grams of carbs and 8 grams of fiber, you can subtract the fiber from the carbs and get the net carbs. So in this case, the apple has 16 net carbs. The fiber slows down the absorption rate of the carbs in your body. For me, it meant that if I ate a bowl of pasta that had 40 grams of carbs and absolutely no fiber, my body would not process the carbs well and my blood sugar level would go up. I would get thirsty and have to go to the bathroom more often. This is a result of the sugar level going up.

Learning just this one thing about carbs and labels has helped me sleep better at night, literally, all because I am not waking up thirsty and having to pee every couple of hours. Leanne and Kelly also taught me about saturated fats, trans fats, hydrogenated and unsaturated fats. I always check the label now to see which fat is in the item I am putting in my cart. What I always choose now is unsaturated fats. Whenever I see any of those other terms, I put it back on the shelf. I don't want to put any food in my mouth that is going to end up clogging my arteries.

The next part of the label I look at is the ingredients list. The ingredients are listed in descending order of the amount in the product. If the first item is sugar, dextrose, or another word for this, then I usually put it back. The more a food is processed, the bigger the words are going to be, and if I can't pronounce it then that is a sure sign that I don't need to put it into my body. I also watch for salt as a main ingredient on the label.

All of this label knowledge has kept me to the perimeters of the store: produce, meat, and dairy sections of the market. Now I very seldom roam up and down the aisles because most of the processed foods are in cans and jars in the middle of the store. I will venture down the frozen food aisle, but I shy away from the fully cooked meals that you just have to heat and eat. I am looking for real food where every bite is going to nurture my body. It is my choice to eat well so I can be healthy. I want every morsel I ingest to bless my body as well as my mind.

I am not saying that I would not have one bite of a brownie if my dear little friend Christopher, who loves to bake, made a pan of them for us. I would take one little bite and savor every last crumb. Here is how this is so very different from my old way of thinking: Before, it was all or nothing. I would totally refuse to eat even one bite because I could not stop at one. Then I would feel like a martyr and begin feeling so sorry for myself. Now I realize that the one bite will keep me from going overboard. I don't have to eat the whole plate of brownies; even a whole plate in the past would not have been enough to fill the empty hole that was inside me. Now I choose to eat one bite and that choice satisfies me more than I can ever express in words. It is all because the Body Clutter that was in my brain and creating those bottomless holes is no longer a threat to my health.

Along with learning to shop more with my brain instead of my taste buds, I have transferred this knowledge to eating in restaurants. We eat out quite often. Robert says that it is better to have a wife who doesn't cook often but can cook, than to have a wife who cooks all the time and can't. I was told by my dear friend Leanne that if I wanted to get rid of my Body Clutter, I was going to have to start cooking. Well, here is one time that I disagree with my personal nutritionist. I can eat out and I can make wise choices. The result for me is that Body Clutter has been decluttered from my thighs. But the weight loss was not my only goal; I was also intent on lowering my blood sugar level.

I have studied the menus of the local restaurants, so now when we venture out to eat I know what choices I have to make. If the restaurant does not have any good choices for my new lifestyle, we stay clear of it. This means that fish and chips are no longer a choice that I would make for myself. Since that was practically the only thing I ate at one of our favorite places, we don't go there anymore. I don't feel deprived because I look carefully at the oil that the fish and fries are cooked in and I choose not to put that in my body. I declutter it before I ever have to deal with it. It is kind of like staying out of stores where you would spend lots of money. I don't choose even to tempt myself by going in the restaurant. Therefore, I don't feel deprived.

Another healthy choice I have made when it comes to eating out is to include a salad made of anything but iceberg lettuce. I usually choose spinach or Romaine lettuce. I ask them to leave off the croutons and put the dressing on the side. This is another little game I play with myself. If I had told them not to give me any dressing, I would have felt deprived. So with the dressing on the side, I can occasionally touch my fork to the top of the bleu cheese. All I needed was to know that I could and I eat only a tiny bit just for the flavor. At the end of the meal, the little container does not even look like I have touched it. I celebrate that I didn't have to eat the whole thing—that I have a choice and I choose to live and enjoy my choices without feeling deprived. The real deprivation would be to leave my sweetie without his life partner. How can I feel deprived when I am making the choice to live a long and healthy life without the complications of obesity and diabetes?

Most restaurants now have low-carb choices on their menus, but if they don't I can still order and ask the waiter for what I want. If I am having salmon, it usually comes with rice. I just have them hold the rice and bring me a serving of steamed broccoli or mixed vegetables. They want our business and it is not being a pain to ask for what you want on your plate. If for some reason I can't request the changes, I just use my empty salad bowl to discard the unhealthy choices and get them off my plate. Then I put a dirty napkin in the bowl. Here is what I know about me: If I leave it on my plate, I will pick at it till it is all gone. This is another form of mindless eating—or, shall I say, my inner brat not wanting to adhere to my choices?

Now for dessert. There is nothing more defeating than being left out while everyone else is having dessert. Even before I made my choice to live, Robert and I were already sharing desserts. It is kind of like have a milk shake with two straws; we just get two forks or spoons. Recently, after an anniversary dinner with friends, the four of us shared a piece of To-Die-For Chocolate Cake. All I wanted was one bite and that was all I needed. We left most of the cake on the plate. We had a lovely dinner with friends. We celebrated their marriage and did not have to feel bad later because of our choices. Many celebrations are fashioned around meals and food. But even in those happy circumstances, we all can learn to make healthy choices for our lives.

We all have to eat, and it is not always about what we choose but when we choose to eat and how much. In the past when I was going to a dinner celebration, I would save up all day. You all know this concept: starve all day and when we get to the celebration, just pig out. We would really act like a hog at those events! That is because we were starving to death. Do you hear this? We had been depriving our body of food all day for the pleasure of eating all we wanted later.

This behavior plays havoc with our metabolism—I dare say Russian roulette because our body has been put into starvation mode all day trying to protect us from a lack of food. Our metabolism slows down. When our metabolism has slowed down to preservation mode, most everything we put in our mouth turns to Body Clutter, perpetuating the cluttered way of thinking that put us bingeing at the buffet table in the first place. Now if I am going to attend a party, I make sure that I eat well all during the day, and that includes my snacks and water, too. Many times about an hour before we leave I eat an apple and a piece of cheese. That keeps me from wanting to stuff everything down my face with a starvation attitude.

We have also learned how not to be too obvious about our eating. When you are grazing, you don't need a plate and, therefore, can't actually keep up with how much you are putting into your body.

The same thing happens at a buffet. We have a great Asian buffet-style restaurant in our town. It has a wonderful salad bar as well as a grill and wok for them to cook your choice of foods. As I have learned to eat on small plates, I turn our trip to the buffet into a several-course meal, but I do not pile my plate up each time I go through the many different buffet lines. I start with a small bowl of soup. Then I pick out two or three pieces of sushi and my favorite condiment, wasabi. Then I may have a small spinach salad. Those are three courses already, and I try to eat them slowly. Then I have them cook my main course or make a wise choice from the buffet tables. By then I am not very hungry and put only a small portion on my plate. There is a dessert bar, too, but by then, I don't even want any dessert.

But if I did, they usually have lots of fresh fruit. My dessert usually consists of my fortune cookie and my cup of hot tea. The waiters keep our water glasses filled throughout the meal, too.

I hope that you can see that every day is made of choices. Our refrigerators reflect the choices we have made in the grocery store. If we don't choose good, healthy food to bring home, we will not have good healthy food to eat when we are home. Learning to make good choices in the grocery store helps you to make the same good choices when you are eating out or at a party. I choose to live! It is just that simple and I don't have to live a deprived life. My choice is a choice of love for me! I love myself enough not to need food to fill that hole any longer.

Not too long ago my sister and I spent time with our ninety-year-old grandmother. She weighs all of eighty pounds. It is not because she does not eat, it is the quality of what she eats. When we looked in her refrigerator, all she had was some milk and snack cakes. She told us that once a week she goes to the grocery store and buys one tray of food from the deli section. She gets ham and two servings of broccoli-and-cheese casserole. She divides this up into three containers and that feeds her the whole week. It is a wonder that she is alive to tell us about this.

The problem was that she could not figure out why she kept losing weight when she was eating. She had no clue that the food she was putting into her body had no nutritional value. Most of it was cooked till all the nutrients were gone. She ate no fresh veggies and filled up on white bread.

No wonder she had a hard time with her bowel movements and had lost the feeling in her fingertips and toes. This is a woman who raised us on a farm, loved fresh vegetables from the garden, and cooked with meat that came from our own land. She has always been a tiny lady, but eighty pounds is not funny. In her mind, food was food. She has since decided to move into an assisted-living facility that allows her still to have her independence but also has people there to help her make better choices.

Isn't that what most of us have always thought? If I just eat something, anything, it will be good enough. That is not the case. We have babies to feed. If we don't know how to feed ourselves, how are we going to know how to feed them?

We are all babies. I am going to take you through the BabySteps of learning about nutrition. This is not rocket science as the media has scared you into thinking. Most of the time we just glaze over whenever we hear about fats and carbs, protein and fiber, and think, I don't have to know this stuff. Yes, we do, if we are going to fill our body with good fuel that gives us the nutrients not just to sustain life but also to help our body function above the bare minimum. Leanne has been working hard to teach me about nutrition. Now I am going to share with you this information in a way that you can understand and not be afraid or intimidated.

We have all heard the expression, "You are what you eat." I want to explain this to you in such a way that you will never again blindly pick up a package of snack cakes without checking the label first. When you make the commitment to put only good fuel in your body, then you will want every bite to have value.

What happens to your car when you put bad gas into it? Oh, it will run most of the time, but it does not give you the necessary power when you need it. Sometimes it is running rough. You know that feeling, too. This is when you can't seem to get going, so you grab a cup of coffee to give you a boost. Did you ever stop to think that this might be a sign from your body that you need fuel and not caffeine? What do you think happens when you grab a snack cake and coffee? This is what Leanne calls "negative nutrition."

I want you to look at a label on a package of food that you have in your pantry. The first thing you see are the words NUTRITION FACTS. And that is what I am going to give you—just the facts, and they are on every packaged product in the grocery store. But if you don't know how to use them, they are in a foreign language to you. Right now you are going to learn not just how to read the label, but to use it as a guide to help you purchase good fuel for your body.

❂ At the top of the label is the **serving size**. Most of us assume that the serving size is the whole package. Keep reading. The label will tell you what the serving size is and how many servings are in the package you are holding. This can be a real shock, especially when we have already eaten the whole thing and are feeling queasy. We have gotten used to megasize servings at restaurants. No wonder we just assume that the package is one serving!

✪ The next part is the **calories per serving** and the **calories from fat per serving**. When these two numbers are very close, that is your first sign that it may not have very many nutrients. But keep reading.

✪ This next section is about the **fats**, **cholesterol**, and **sodium** that are in one serving of the packaged product. I know this can be confusing, which is why I want to enlighten you. There are four types of fats. I am going to start with saturated fat. It is good to limit these to very small amounts.

✪ **Saturated fat** mainly comes from animals: meat, milk, eggs, cheese. There are a few plant oils that are saturated, too: palm and coconut. For the most part, these fats are solid at room temperature. Think about lard. It is made from animal fat. These fats raise our bad cholesterol. If you eat lots of this kind of fat, you are clogging your arteries. That is why we want you to limit the quantity of saturated fats in the food you put in your mouth.

✪ The next fat is **monounsaturated fat**. This comes from plants. It is a good fat, but as with any good thing, too much can hurt you. So it is a good idea to make sure that each bite you take has less than 30 percent fat. Since good fat should be part of eating, plant fat is the one to eat. Limit your saturated fats and supplement them with an unsaturated fat. Here is a list of foods that contain monounsaturated fat: olives, olive oil, almonds, peanuts, other nuts, seeds, and avocados. We want to teach you about balance in all things and that includes fats. A monounsaturated fat is good for your arteries. It does not increase your bad cholesterol and it does not reduce your good cholesterol.

We do need some fat to help our body digest nutrients. Since we will be eating some fat, we might as well make it good for us at the same time, but be sure to pick a monounsaturated fat. This is a healthy choice. A polyunsaturated fat has many of the same good qualities as the monounsaturated fats. All fats have the same amount of calories, so it is wise to keep fat consumption to as little as possible.

✪ Now here is the one fat that is definitely *not* a good choice. As you would tell your babies, this is a no-no! A **trans fat** started out life as a good fat but has been hydrogenated, which has to do with its chemical molecular structure. They have taken a fat that is liquid at room temperature and changed its structure to a solid at room temperature. They have done this to increase its shelf life and make it not break down in frying. This fat has been linked to coronary heart disease and clogged arteries. This is also true of partially hydrogenated fats, which are contained in many packaged products. They are so bad that the government is requiring foods that contain them to say so on the label. Stay as far away from them as possible.

What have you learned at this point by looking at the label? If the level of fat makes up almost half of its calories, then it may not be a good choice. If the fat in the food is trans fat, then it is your choice to reduce your life by eating it. I know this may sound harsh, but it is really that simple. We should not be putting trans fat in our body. Eating deep-fried foods is not a good selection at a restaurant. If the food you are eating has less than 30 percent fat, then it is a good choice, but only in small quantities. If you are eating meat, pick the leanest cuts. Right now we are learning how to decipher those labels and utilize this knowledge to feed our families well.

I have found out a trade secret of the manufacturers. If they take out the fat, they have to add something back to give the food some flavor. It is usually sodium or sugar.

❂ The next item on the label is **cholesterol**. This will tell you how many milligrams of cholesterol are in the food. Your liver already makes cholesterol, so any you eat is added to what your body is already making. A healthy person should not be eating more than 300 milligrams of cholesterol per day. An egg yolk has 214 milligrams. When you look at a label, it will tell you what percent of your daily allowance this food will give you. If the percentage is high, it means that this serving is just about all you should have of cholesterol in one day. Combine that with the other foods you have already eaten and you get the picture. We don't eat just this one thing. We have to think about everything on our plate as well as our daily food consumption to make sure we are not going overboard with this section of the label.

✷ Now we come to **sodium**. This is salt. If we eat too much salt we start to retain water and get puffy fingers. The daily allowance for a healthy person is 2,400 milligrams. This is the total amount of salt for the day. Divide that by three meals and three snacks and you can see just how far it will go. Now go to your refrigerator and find a package of cheese. See the amount of sodium in just one string cheese. It is 280 milligrams. Now this is not bad, but you cannot eat seven of them. That is one reason why you should eat a balanced diet, spreading out your daily allowance to cover all your meals and your snacks.

✷ To the right of all the grams and milligrams you will see percentages. This number tells you what part this serving of food is of your daily allotment of 2,000 calories— that is, if you are eating 2,000 calories. Now, remember, to get rid of Body Clutter you are going to have to eat less than you have been and move more. When you are looking at any food label (the top section), you need to keep the numbers small (grams and percentages). The total calorie consumption per day varies for each person.

The average adult who has no major weight issues generally should consume approximately 2,000 calories per day. A person trying to lose Body Clutter would often be recommended to eat fewer than 2,000. Please check with your doctor to find out the appropriate caloric intake for you.

✿ The next section is what I have to look at all the time. Not a single bite goes in my mouth unless I know how many **carbohydrates** it has in it. I love carbs—you name it: bread, pasta, rice, dessert, and my sweet tea and lemonade. These food labels have been so helpful for my new diabetic lifestyle.

Let me explain to you what a carbohydrate is. This is a food that when put into our body is either sugar, or your digestion process (also known as metabolizing) turns it into sugar. If the truth be known, all food eventually turns into sugar. This is what gives our body energy. It is the speed at which the food becomes sugar that causes our babies to bounce off the wall when they have binged on candy.

This is what happens to our blood sugar: It takes a huge jump almost immediately when we ingest liquid sugar in soft drinks and sweet foods. It also happens when we eat white flour, rice, and potatoes. Do you remember, as a child in school, your teacher giving you a cracker to chew and chew? We could not swallow it; we just had to keep chewing. Eventually it went from tasting salty to tasting sweet. That is how our digestion works. Our bodies convert the starch into a sugar. Bread, rice, and potatoes are starches and they convert rapidly into sugar.

If the label says it has 24 grams of carbohydrates, it means that it is the equivalent of 6 teaspoons of sugar. Just put that in your coffee and stir it! A soft drink has a little more than this amount—how does 40 grams of sugar sound to you? That is ten teaspoons of sugar. Every teaspoon is 15 calories. The carbohydrate section of a label tells us about the fiber and the added sugar.

❂ The **fiber grams** reduce the carbs by the same amount. That is because the fiber slows down the absorption rate of the sugar by the body. Fiber also helps our body to eliminate the food residue that cannot be used. This is good for our colon. We need 25 grams of fiber a day.

❂ Our body needs **protein** to build muscle. Adult women need 45 to 50 grams of protein each day. It is good for us to choose lean protein to keep our fat consumption to a minimum. Think of meat, and other proteins, as a garnish for your plate or sandwich. A little goes a long way. If you like to have a piece of meat on your plate at dinner, then you are going to have to eat like a vegetarian during the day. You can get protein in more than just meat. Think about fish, beans, nuts, and milk products.

❂ Next I want you to look at the very bottom of the label. This section is for the **vitamin** content in the food. This will tell you whether the food you are putting into your body has any redeeming nutritional value. It will tell you what percentage of your daily requirements for each vitamin is in each serving.

I know this is boring stuff, but feeding yourself and your family is worth a little studying so you will know what you are doing. Knowledge is power, and the sooner we educate ourselves to have the power over our Stinking Thinking, the sooner we will have begun to release the Body Clutter from between our ears to create a new way of life for ourselves and our loved ones.

## Body Clutter Mission

Open your Body Clutter Control Journal to a blank page. Now go to your pantry and look at the packages.

Make a list of all the food that has trans fat listed on the nutrition label.

Are any of these your comfort foods?

What voices do you hear when you sit down to eat?

Were you forced to join the "Clean Plate Club"?

Do you have vegetables that you will not allow in your home now because you had to sit for hours till you had eaten them, hidden those Brussels sprouts or butter beans, or fed them to the dog?

Now think about what you may have done to your children nutritionally. This is the hard part. Forgive yourself. Don't beat yourself up over this. We don't have to be perfect. We are educating and forgiving ourselves. This is all part of getting rid of our Body Clutter!

# 9. Moving

Perspective is everything when it comes to what qualifies as moving. Your perspective and mine could be completely different, but the bottom line is making sure there is indeed some movement going on with your body. For some people, parking your car farther out in the parking lot at the grocery store can be a good place to get started; for other people, there is a need for more than that.

*Leanne*

I was one of those people who just couldn't get things going till I made a serious commitment to getting physically fit. It's as if a light went on for me—not everyone does everything the same! This is so basic and yet it eluded me forever! My way isn't FlyLady's way and neither is mine hers. The issue was that we both needed movement in our lives. I am dealing with a thyroid condition and FlyLady is dealing with diabetes. While we are not defining ourselves by our diseases, based on my research, I was going to have to really get going in order to get the Body Clutter off.

Still, my intention was to do as little as possible—I was willing to do only the bottom-line minimum. However, I desperately wanted to incorporate movement into my daily routine, so I tried doing the extra steps. I tried walking and videos and all that stuff, but it wasn't doing anything for me because I had not made it the priority that it had to be for me to get healthy—and I was more frustrated than ever. So to make a long story short, it wasn't long before my "movement" became full-on, hard-core exercise. I know that sounds just awful and sweaty and not at all fun. However, I would ask your indulgence just to hang in there with me and hear my story.

There comes a point in everyone's life when you have to make decisions you would rather not. It wasn't that I was lazy or had an injury or anything, it was just overwhelming to look at all that needed doing. I mean, I was well over two-hundred pounds and while I was pretty unhappy with the state of my body, I was unhappier with the idea of having to go through the unpleasant task of "working out." Once again, that perfectionism was front and center. I believe perfectionism wants us to look at all that needs to be done, overwhelms us with how hard it is, and then the negative self-talk starts. To me, this is a critical part of Body Clutter—it's not just on our hips but also between our ears. We talk to ourselves and pull ourselves down before we even get started! This is how we create a very personal pattern. We did that with our messy house and we do that with our personal house (our body). Too overwhelming, too much work, we start to whine, we start to look for excuses, and we rationalize why we're there in the first place. I wasn't looking at the right stuff—I was looking at the finished product, and by not embracing the process by Baby-Stepping and focusing on just doing something, I was defeated before I started.

But I had to face the facts—FlyLady's wake-up call was also mine. I was of the opinion that God wasn't messing around and it was critical to look at the reality of the situation, assess what needed to be done, and *then* put my efforts into the BabySteps. Do you see the difference? I still made a big-picture analysis, but because of BabySteps did it without the paralysis of no action. God bless BabySteps! So the big-picture analysis was simple: I was going to have to get my Franny moving to get that Body Clutter off me.

I made a financial decision to invest in my health. If there is something I don't know enough about, I'm going to find an expert to help me. Consequently, I hired a personal trainer and made it my goal just to show up. That was my first BabyStep: showing up! I know that sounds dumb, but for me it's how I started to declutter some of the Stinking Thinking that had held me back for so many years.

Now, I know there are a lot of people who would roll their eyes at the hiring of a personal trainer and maybe even call it frivolous. I look at it in a much different way and consider the true frivolity I've "invested" in—junk food, diet scams, books, and pills. That was serious cash completely lost with nothing to show for it. No, wait, I take that back. I did have something to show for the junk food and I was sitting on it. Years ago, personal trainers were something that only the rich and famous could afford and utilize. Now there are personal trainers at most gyms to help you get started. Some places offer a few sessions for free with a membership or even offer a free evaluation for just walking through the door. Don't be afraid of what you think may be too expensive without some research.

After the first week of working out with this guy, sitting in a chair and standing up hurt! I was convinced I was doing too much. I definitely felt the burn! But I hung in there anyway (with the help of ibuprofen and prayer!) and got through the hardest part. The sessions themselves were only a half-hour long. My perfectionism, of course, rolled itself back out and I wondered if "only a half hour" would be "enough." I decided to keep at it, however, and soon discovered it was indeed enough. It was hard! Yet, because of the way the exercises are set up in the session, I was able to cheerlead myself on, "Go, Me!" I took each exercise as it came and BabyStepped all the way, challenging myself to do "just one more." I was shocked at how easily I adapted to this new routine, and within a month had easily dropped ten pounds of Body Clutter! ME! The girl with the problem thyroid and perfectionist attitude dropped ten without even blinking!

One warm spring day I was driving in the car. I was wearing a short-sleeved T-shirt and listening to the radio.

The light turned red, I stopped, and as a matter of habit, extended my right arm out straight to the steering wheel. As I was waiting for the light to turn, I looked over to the right and didn't recognize my own arm. There was *muscle* in it and it looked good! Where once there was flab, there was now muscle and definition! I was positively thrilled. The feeling was one of amazing empowerment—I felt strong and in control of my own body. I will never forget that day as long as I live.

Remember when you were little and you had an insatiable curiosity and sense of wonder? You would lie in the grass with your friends for hours gazing at the clouds in the sky, watching one cloud turn from a dragon to a dog to an angel. You would spend your afternoons picking clover flowers and make clover crowns for your heads. You would run with wild abandon and try to capture butterflies and lizards. The whole world was your oyster and you were BabyStepping all over the place, filling your senses with how wonderful and magnificent it all was. There was a sense of awe in your world.

There is a similar sense of wonder that happens to you as your body starts to change. It feels just like it did when you were little—school was out, it was summer, and you were allowed to play outside till the streetlights came on. There was a feeling of freedom, a feeling of no constraints.

These little lightbulbs and moments of recognition were starting to happen on a regular basis and I was discovering a whole new world. I noticed that my moods of highs and lows were evening out and I was happier with the world around me. But one of the biggest lights to go on was that becoming physically fit truly meant something to me that I was never able to realize before. I started to love myself enough to value the body that God had given me. FLYing had become more multidimensional than ever before. I had missed that part of FLYing until then.

My body is by no means perfect—I've got stretch marks on my tummy from giving birth to two large babies. I've got spider veins on the back of my legs, and my boobs certainly aren't as perky as they were when I was twenty, but I had started to recover my body and I found out that I liked it! The harder I worked, the more I wanted to push myself and the more I enjoyed the ride. Another lightbulb went on: I wanted to challenge myself to do something that I had never done before; I wanted to run a 5-K race. Without those BabySteps and routines there is no way that I would have ever considered challenging myself to do that.

Although I was an avowed hater of anything even resembling running, it was during one of those thirty-minute sessions with my trainer that I started to run. We'd work out with the weights for a little while, and then he'd throw me on the treadmill and make me run for two minutes. The first time I did it, I was complaining the whole time. "I can't run, Joe! Don't make me run. I'll walk fast, but no running." He kept it up, and in no time I was completely surprised at how it had become easier and easier to accomplish.

The week before my forty-seventh birthday, I decided I wanted to run a 5-K. No particular reason why, except to say I did it. It was a new goal for me. This is again where we are all different; some of us don't like to have a "goal" hanging over our heads, and some of us need that goal to keep us motivated. We all march to the beat of our own drum and that is okay. Ultimately, living our lives to be healthy through the BabySteps that we establish is what is important. I've always liked having goals to help me track where I'm going— I've done this more or less my whole life, but the physical side of goal setting wasn't anything I was used to. It was thrilling, too, being able to take something I used to hate and turn it into something I love! Well, maybe that's a stretch. I still do not love running, but I don't loathe it either, and that's a quantum leap up from where I started, that is for sure.

For now, I am able to run a mile without stopping. I'm still in training for my 5-K and will be running my first one soon. I know without a shadow of a doubt that had I not started to take my health seriously and understand the importance of being physically fit, this wouldn't have happened.

Another thing that I discovered was the strong correlation between your house and your body. Your body is your most private house. It houses the soul. This is the place where the internal conversations happen—truly, where you "live." Your house is your environment, and the reflection of its visual order (or disorder) hugely affects the conversations that happen inside your most private house—your body. I hope this makes sense; this was an important discovery for me.

When I finally got my house in order, via BabySteps and routines, the first thing I wanted to do was decorate. There I was with this great house that looked awful. So I started to decorate—new paint went on the walls, I hung curtains and pictures, the whole nine yards. My newly decluttered house became a warm, cozy home because I had spent the time and energy to make it so. Think about what this means for your body. When you declutter your body, the first thing you want to do is decorate as well. That often means a new haircut, some makeup perhaps, new clothes to flatter your changing body. You don't have to have a lot of money to "redecorate," just a few ideas to make your home your own. And when you're redecorating that most personal home (your body), it can be an absolute blast! Nothing is more thrilling than trying on clothes in your previous size to find they are too big!

But there are obstacles along the way to that place of decorating. I found that the biggest obstacle I had to face was *me*. I was the deterrent and the antagonist. But when I let go of the perfectionism and Stinking Thinking and was open to the possibilities, amazing things began to happen and today I hardly even recognize myself anymore. I don't mean just physically, I mean healthwise, as well as mentally and emotionally. My cholesterol is low, my skin looks one-hundred times better, I think more clearly, my emotions are in check (no PMS!), and I am happy being me.

It's been very hard and a lot of work to get here, and I'm still working at it! Even if I reach my goal weight, I will always be a work in progress. This is the process of releasing our Body Clutter—it doesn't end with a goal weight; it's a lifestyle change that completely reenergizes your life and changes the way you think. To me, there is nothing like waking up every morning, throwing on your running shorts, and hitting the road—even if you have to walk and run, like I do. Being able to enjoy the ability to move and run and see nature along the way has done more for my peace of mind than just about anything else. Who knew?

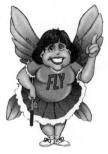

FlyLady

I have been trying to figure out why I have never liked to exercise—and I do have some clues. In school, gym class was where I was ridiculed for not being very coordinated. I have always been aerobically challenged. The sad part was that in school they did not teach us that moving was an important part of our overall health. All I learned was exercise equals punishment. Even if I was not forced to run laps or do push-ups, exercise class was always torture.

As an adult going back to college, I had to sign up for a physical education class. That really scared me, so I picked a dance-aerobics class as my PE credit. Three times a week I had to attend an 8 A.M. class and learn an aerobic routine. Let's just say, the nicest way to put it is that I had two left feet. I felt completely out of place with the college kids who all seemed to know every movement. The instructor just glided through the routine while I flubbed up every step, not being able to clap my hands and kick my feet at the same time. Most days I left the class practically in tears. By the end of the semester I got an award for being the most-improved aerobically challenged student. Imagine that: I got an award for not being perfect. I finally figured out that I didn't have to be the best at it to get credit for the class. I just needed to show up, keep moving, and learn to laugh at myself.

Showing up is half the battle that takes place in our head. Once we get started with anything, it is never as bad as we have talked ourselves into believing it was going to be. So we might as well "Just Do It" as the Nike commercial says. The funny thing about moving is that we always feel better when we finish. We no longer have the guilt for not doing it and we have blessed our bodies by moving. The best thing is that as moving becomes an automatic part of our daily routine, we don't even have to think about it. Eventually, we actually look forward to our daily body-blessing ritual.

We have to make choices every day. Moving and blessing our body is another choice we can make. We can choose to be a slug and feel like a sack of pennies, or we can take BabySteps to get off our Frannies and get the blood pumping through our veins.

We don't have to beat ourselves up any longer because we need to get in shape. If the truth be told, most of us have never been, and will never be, as fit as an Olympic athlete. If your choice is to live a long and healthy life, it is not going to be done sitting on the sidelines watching the world FLY by. We have to get up and join the parade!

All our lives we have been trying to save our steps and save time in the process. But are we truly saving time, or are we really robbing ourselves of precious days on this earth with our families? I want you to think about searching for the closest parking place at the mall; we have all done it. I have even thanked the "angel of parking" for allowing one to open up right at the front door. Now I am wondering if my thanks were given to the proper recipient. Maybe it was the "angel of death" who opened up that parking place just so I would make it to the cemetery sooner.

My attitude has changed when it comes to taking extra steps. I now look for ways to enjoy my journey and not get there as fast as I can. My timer is set and every 15 minutes during the day I get off my Franny and move. I don't have to do much, just get up and get the blood flowing in my legs. The more I move, the more I want to move. It is as contagious as a shiny sink.

With my new attitude I look forward to my thirty minutes of aerobic activity three days a week. I am not beating myself up because I am not doing five days a week yet. I know that as I get stronger I will work out more often and for longer periods of time. I am already feeling the desire to take another BabyStep to bless my heart an additional day each week. Here is what I know about me: If I go hog wild, I will crash and burn and it will happen before I can ever establish my new habit. I choose to live, and this choice takes into account my all-or-nothing attitude. I need BabySteps to protect myself from my perfectionism. I also need to make any kind of moving I do fun. If it is not fun or I feel awkward and punished, I will not want to do it. I have found that I need variety to spice up my moving.

Part of my new attitude about moving and blessing my heart comes from letting go of the bad things that have happened to me, my little insecurities, and stepping out in faith that I can do this. It doesn't have to be perfect. My choice is life! It is just that simple. I can either watch my life wither away for lack of use, or I can prevent the atrophy by getting up and moving.

You know what they say, "If you don't use it, you will lose it." I don't want to lose my life because I was just too unmotivated to get up and start. Life is too short as it is. As I have been moving more, I have noticed that my energy level has increased. I now accept that moving is an important part of my overall wellness, and refusing to do it doesn't hurt anyone but me.

When we rebel against moving we are only condemning ourselves to a shorter lifetime of inactivity. I believe the reason that we refuse to move has more to do with punishment. So let's remove that aspect and celebrate every moment of movement.

Maybe you are taking your sweet puppy out for a walk every day. But instead of just getting his business done, you give your puppy an energizing walk around the block. Your dog is happy and your body is saying, "Go Me!" Your critter will begin to anticipate your putting on your moving shoes. For me, I need a buddy to get me up and out of my chair. A dear friend and I have a standing appointment—actually a moving appointment—every Monday, Wednesday, and Friday to get together to move and cheer each other on. We depend on each other to motivate ourselves. When she is unable to do a move, I encourage her, and when I am not able, she gives me the boost that I need. Before we know it we have completed a thirty-minute aerobic video and we are celebrating.

Moving has to be incorporated into your daily routine. Some people like to get their moving done when they first get up in the morning. I am often asked, "Do I have to get up and get dressed to shoes only to get sweaty and have to take another shower in order to begin my day?" The answer to this question is quite simple: It depends on your personal daily schedule. If you do your moving first thing, you can just shower after that; if not, two showers can be twice as nice.

Lay out two sets of clothes for yourself each evening: your cute workout clothes and the clothes you are going to wear after you work out. If you are headed to work in the morning, you will need to do your Morning Routine along with getting out the door to the gym. Your clothes and makeup for work are packed in a bag that you put together the night before, and in the morning you dress for the gym. You will have two routines that merge into one another as your day begins.

When your feet first hit the floor, there is only one thing on your mind—to Bless Your Heart. You immediately dress for your movement time. But don't allow yourself to skip your Morning Routine because FlyLady told you to move. You just have to piggyback this onto what you are already successfully doing. If your home goes back to the chaotic shape it was in, you will not feel like you have the time to move. So let go of your all-or-nothing perfectionist attitude and merge these two routines. I like to think about this as learning a new dance step.

We have gotten the Before Bed Routine down pat. Then we add laying out another set of clothes. Now when your feet hit the floor in the morning, you are all gung-ho on your new moving routine, but you can't throw out what you have been doing for months just because you feel this is more important now. You have to blend them together to fit your home and your schedule. We are building on good foundations, not tearing down old routines and replacing them with new ones that omit creating a peaceful home. When your home is a mess, then so are you. Your home is just a symptom of what is going on inside you. Don't allow it to overshadow your successes in the Body Clutter arena by tearing down the peace you have established.

Back to that dance step. When you learn to do one part you can easily add another one till you have built your routines, one BabyStep after another. We have to practice them each day. But if we try to do too much too fast, you know what will happen. We will crash and burn, and then we feel worse than before we started. We don't want this to happen, but it does. So when it does, I just want you to jump back in where you are and continue to celebrate your successes and not whine over your messing up. It is the consistency of doing it every day that is going to reinforce this new habit for you.

I have included my routine for moving as part of my afternoon routine three days a week. At 3 P.M. we meet at my house or at our office to spend thirty minutes in an aerobic activity. We have several aerobic DVDs to choose from. I usually come home and hop into the shower after a sweaty workout. You have to adapt your routine to fit your personal schedule. The main thing I want you to remember is that your routine is not complete till you have changed out of your workout clothes and put on your regular clothes. I know your workout clothes may be cute, but you have to take a shower and get dressed. You cannot stay in your workout clothes all day.

There is another important aspect of movement that I want you to think about. There have been times in all of our lives that we have been depressed in some way. Just the simple act of getting up and moving for 15 minutes is good for our mental health as well as our physical health. The activity releases chemicals in our brain that make us feel better about ourselves. I don't know exactly what happens, but maybe it could be that the simple act of loving ourselves makes us have a feeling of peace.

For years I have taught others that when you put a smile on your face it tells your head that you are happy. That little muscle movement in your face creates the feeling of being happy. Isn't it the feeling of peace that we are searching for? Just like our lace-up shoes tell our head that it is time to go to work, our workout clothes and a little loving movement can go a long way in helping us to release the dark cloud that has been following us. Let's lace up those shoes and see just how good we can feel about ourselves—body, mind and, most of all, spirit!

Your calendar, your timer, and even your feather duster can help to motivate you. Reward yourself with a cute sticker, a heart, or a star on your calendar each time you Bless Your Heart. Soon you will begin to see your routine take shape right along with your Body Clutter melting away. Use your timer because, as always, you can do anything for 15 minutes, even Bless Your Heart. My duster has become a tool for my work out. I feel just like a cheerleader holding it in my hand to do my aerobics. I love cheering myself on! Find a reason to celebrate. Chart your success and, most of all, have fun at what you are doing. If it is fun, you will do it!

**Make It Fun!**

So how can we make moving fun for us? First, by letting go of our perfectionism and that internal need to compete with some imaginary foe. Moving is not a battle to the death; it is a habit we are practicing to help us live long and healthy lives. If we start out trying to kill ourselves to get in "shape" we will not stick with our moving routines. It becomes too hard. We can't live up to our perfectionism. One way we can make moving fun is to find something that we like to do: dancing, walking, swimming, aerobics, yoga, tai chi, gardening, fly-fishing, hiking, etc. If you're not sure, think back to when you were a child and the activities that you liked to do then.

I remember spending hours in the creek, hiking for miles just playing in the water. Guess what I enjoy doing now?

Fly-fishing and hiking up a creek for hours. Not only am I blessing my body by moving, but I also get lost in a calm meditation while I am there. The trouble with fly-fishing is I don't do it every day. I still need to move on a daily basis, so how can I find something else that makes me feel good? Since I live in a wooded area, I can take a short walk in my woods or get on my treadmill that is surrounded by windows with bird feeders. I can also go outside and pull weeds in my garden. That uses muscles when I'm bending and stretching. You don't even realize you are moving when you are having a good time—the time FLYs when you are having fun.

As perfectionists we get stuck in our Stinking Thinking. We think we need to spend an hour exercising and getting our heart rate up to those levels that our former aerobics instructor demanded of us. Our fear of not doing it right keeps us couch potatoes. If we push ourselves too hard too fast, we don't do anything. Isn't a little moving better than no moving at all? We have to learn to take BabySteps to increase our activity levels and not beat ourselves up because we are not doing it the "right way." After all, just 15 minutes a day can change the way you feel about yourself.

Sometimes we just need to play a game with ourselves to increase our moving. Wearing a pedometer will show you just how many steps you take in a day. Every step is moving, isn't it? It doesn't matter if you are not on some exercise regimen. We can add a few more steps each day by not driving around looking for a parking space at the front door of Wal-Mart. Find reasons to walk: Park at the end of the lot, take the stairs when you usually take the elevator, or walk down your driveway to pick up your mail. We are not trying to save steps anymore; let's increase them so we can move just a little more—and we won't even realize it. And best of all, we are blessing our body at the same time.

There are days that I just cannot wait to get out of bed and get on the treadmill. One day in particular I wanted to get on that treadmill and I wanted to write! For some reason I had words burning my fingertips and then the phone rang. It was Kelly, and I wanted to speak with her, so I decided to try something new that morning. I got on the treadmill and talked to her at the same time. Let's just say that it is much easier for me to walk and type than it is to walk and talk. Go figure! But I did it! I can do a lot of things with my phone. I have one of those headset phones that clip on my waistband and it looks like the phone is surgically implanted in my head. You won't believe what I can get done with this phone on my head. I have done interviews and pulled weeds at the same time. One of my favorite things to do on the phone is grab my feather duster and dance around the house while I am talking. My hands are free and I don't even realize that I am cleaning. Now, my husband thinks I look like an alien, but my headset phone is one of my favorite tools for making moving fun!

I hope you are beginning to see that if we make it fun, it will get done. We love fun and games. If what we do is not fun, it seems too much like work and we will just put it off! That is another reason I use my timer all the time. I don't have to think, it thinks for me! A timer is an excellent tool to

BabyStep your way to Blessing Your Heart. You can give yourself permission to set the timer and you have to move only for the time that you set. If it is only five minutes of walking, that is five minutes more than what you were doing. BabyStepping your way to Blessing Your Heart is the best gift you can give to yourself.

## Create a Special Place for Finally Loving Yourself

There is no specific day or time that we have to choose to start FLYing in order to address our Body Clutter. We don't have to wait for a new year to decide to take care of ourselves. We only have to make the choice that today will be the day that I will love myself enough to take care of me. What do we mean when we decide to FLY? It all boils down to a lifestyle change for many of us. Now, we could go cold turkey and go away for a month to some elaborate spa where they fix our meals for us, put us on an exercise regimen, run medical tests, and pamper us, or we can learn from them and do it ourselves. We can create our very own spa at home.

If you went away to one of those retreats for a month, what would be the first thing they would do to you? You would have to sign a waiver and get a physical and blood work. Why do you think they make you sign a waiver? It is to relinquish them from any liability that could result from your keeling over from a heart attack. This in itself should be a wake-up call for most of us. Our lifestyles are contributing to the increase of obesity, heart disease, and diabetes. With this in mind, it is up to each one of us to take charge of our body and our mind and go get a physical along with the blood work. We should do this before we start any new lifestyle changes. This is the barometer to help guide us. Do not procrastinate about this. Make your appointment today because this is the first step to the rest of your life. Talk to your doctor about taking BabySteps to change your life. Ask for help and, as long as you are getting blood work done, get them to run a full-panel thyroid screen. Do not allow your perfectionism, or your fears, to creep in and keep you from getting a physical.

At the spa you would probably be forced to go cold turkey when it comes to smoking, alcohol, and caffeine. How can we limit these things for ourselves while we are enjoying our home spa? Let's look realistically at how much we are doing these things during a day, week, or month, as well as how much money they cost us. For some people, saving money can be a motivating factor. Others just decide that moderation is the key. Instead of five cups of coffee a day, have just one. Then replace each missing cup of coffee with a bottle of water. With dinner have water and one glass of wine instead of a bottle. Be nice to yourself and don't punish yourself by taking everything away cold turkey, which is what most fad diets require. You know how well that works! You feel deprived and then you just throw the diet out the window and devour all you can get your hands on.

Smoking is a very hard habit to break, so look at when your body is craving a cigarette and when it is just a simple habit to light up. You will be able to tell the difference and start eliminating them, one BabyStep at a time.

We can turn our homes into nurturing spas with just a few little additions to our grocery lists. Spas have good wholesome snacks just waiting for you to enjoy them. They require you to eat several times during the day. We don't normally do that because we are too busy to eat. The main reason we don't eat good, wholesome foods is that there aren't any in the refrigerator. Add whole fruits, cut-up veggies, nuts, cottage cheese cups, yogurt, and salad fixings to your weekly grocery list. Remind yourself to eat between meals. Imagine that—you have permission to snack!

At a spa you never see anyone without a water bottle. There are water coolers everywhere and little reminders to drink up. I am not talking about overdoing it here, just getting eight glasses of water a day. If you eat three meals a day and three snacks a day, and drink a small glass with each, then you have had six glasses of water. Now add one when you get up while you are getting dressed and then another one before bed. You have done it—eight glasses in a sixteen-hour day. That is only one glass every couple of hours. Set your timer if you have to so you will remember to drink your water.

Now for the hard part of being at a spa! They are going to force you to get into shape. We have been couch potatoes for a very long time, but now we have given "them" permission to help us. Let's give ourselves this same permission. You may need to ask a friend to help you. It is much easier if you have someone whom you are accountable to. Not moving is not an option; the spa trainer is not going to accept any excuse for your inactivity. Moving can be as simple as walking around your yard or on a treadmill. Start by adding a 15-minute walk to your Morning Routine. Then gradually you will be incorporating other BabySteps to your daily walk through life. Little things like parking farther from the front door at the grocery store or taking the stairs whenever you can. Before you know it you will be playing in the yard with the children or taking the dog for a romp, having a great time incorporating loving movement into your everyday life. When you make it fun, it will continue to Bless Your Heart.

A spa has lots of ways to pamper you, starting with your bedroom. The beds are nice and inviting. They encourage you to go to bed at a decent hour by having a curfew. When was the last time you went to bed before 11 P.M.? There are fresh sheets on your bed and plump pillows to curl up on with a good book for a few minutes of leisuretime. Getting rest is one of the keys to helping our body renew itself and heal. There have been studies that correlate obesity to not getting enough sleep. Go to bed and quit making your body beg for sleep. Our body needs good food, water, loving movement, and rest to function properly.

We also need to reward ourselves for the simple life changes we are making. At our home spa we can do things like manicures, pedicures, bubble baths, facials, and other little things to help us feel good about the BabySteps we are making part of our routines. These little rewards help you feel good about you and teach you to FLY (Finally Love Yourself), and isn't that what Blessing Your Heart is all about? We deserve to live happy, healthy, productive lives. Enjoy your spa!

## The Basic Weekly Plan

It is one thing to talk about moving, but I also want to motivate you into getting off your Franny to Bless Your Heart. Important things to do before you start any moving routine:

1. Check with your doctor first.
2. Lay out your moving clothes along with your regular clothes the night before. Don't forget your shoes.
3. Drink your water.
4. Take the babies along in the stroller if you have little ones.
5. Take BabySteps. Do not overdo it and crash and burn. Start slow and steady. You can even do a little in the morning and a little in the afternoon and gradually do a little more as it gets easier.
6. After you move, put a star on your calendar to chart your progress.

The FlyLady system has a Basic Weekly Plan for our home. We use this plan for cleaning our home, getting ready for the holidays, and our work schedule. We can implement this plan to incorporate our loving movements, so that moving is a normal part of our daily life. Let's look at our Basic Weekly Plan for moving.

❂ **Monday is Home Blessing Day**. Take a few minutes on Monday also to bless your body with an energizing workout. You could walk at a faster pace or do an aerobic videotape. Start out taking BabySteps. Do not overdo it. Set your timer.

- **Tuesday is Free Day**. This doesn't mean that you don't have to move; think about it as freestyle! Do something off the wall: Dance to some music, march to the beat of a different drum or, while sitting down on the job, do some slow stretches. You are very creative. I have seen everything from hula hoops to trampolines.

- **Wednesday is always Anti-Procrastination Day!** Combine your moving with something you have been putting off. It could be that you need to touch base with a friend. Call her up and meet to go walking. If you can't meet in person, take your cell phone along and put on your headset so you can keep your arms moving.

- **Thursday is Errand Day!** Since you have to be out anyway, why not park your car in the last space in the parking lot and take a few extra minutes to walk to the store, or walk around the mall a couple of times before you start your shopping.

- **Friday is our Date Night!** Take a walk with your sweetie or do an activity that you both love. We go bowling, and let me tell you—you can get a pretty good workout throwing a bowling ball! If you are single, set this date on your calendar as a day for you to enjoy yourself with your friends. Don't sit home in front of the TV, eating bonbons and feeling sorry for yourself. Take the first BabyStep to connect with your close friends.

- **Saturday is Family Fun Day!** Plan a hike or a day in the park to play! Spend it with your family and enjoy the outdoors. Look in the newspaper for festivals and enjoy the day walking. In the summer, go for a swim or a bike ride. You can find lots of things to do as a family if you just think about it a little. Remember that your family does not always have to be people you are related to. Many families are made up of close friends.

❂ **Sunday is always Renew Your Spirit Day!** As part of this day, take a few minutes to take a walk either on your treadmill listening to wonderful music or in your favorite area outside.

See how easy it is to incorporate moving in your Basic Weekly Plan?

## Body Clutter Mission

In your Body Clutter Control Journal, turn to another clean sheet of paper. We are going to get honest about just how sedentary we are. Be aware that perfectionism is going to try to keep you from writing.

When was the last time you worked up a sweat moving? What were you doing? Write it down!

Do you have a good pair of lace-up athletic shoes? When was the last time you bought a new pair? Old shoes will cause injury. Your homework assignment is to go get your foot measured at an athletic-shoe store. Now write down what you think your shoe size is, and when you get back write down what the store said.

# 10. Attitude

_Leanne_

Patti LaBelle sang a song years ago called "New Attitude." Part of the lyrics to the chorus go, "I'm feeling good from my head to my shoes, know where I'm going and know what to do, oo oo oo oo oooo, I've got a new attitude!" Can't help but wonder with the reference to shoes if she is a Fly-Baby! Interesting, too, how she felt good from her head to her shoes and knew what to do—is that what FLYing is about or _what_?

We are given so many choices in life—we can whine and complain or we can get off our duff and get honest with ourselves as in, "This isn't working—what can I do differently?" Our attitude is our choice. It's either a good one that blesses our families, or a stinky one that reeks and smells up the whole house. You choose—it's your choice. In the past, we've all been given some awful Christmas or birthday gift that we truly didn't want. Some of us had the privilege of exchanging the clunker for a gem, and others had to haul it off with the rest of the clutter in our homes. Either way, getting rid of something through an exchange or dumping makes way for an upgrade in our lives.

That's how it is with our attitude toward whatever it is that we're doing. We have a choice of how we're going to approach things in our lives. You can't just expect your life to take care of itself when you do nothing about it. I promise you, complaining doesn't do a thing, it just draws attention to the fact that you're a whiner and that's the only action you're willing to throw at your problems. You're certainly not hitting a lick at a snake when all you do is whine.

But with a new attitude in place, the world is your oyster. Hope replaces despair, "I can't" is replaced with "I will." A willingness and softness of heart to change your mind and even admit you're wrong is a far better choice than a martyred attitude, anger, and bitterness toward someone else—or yourself.

How easily this overlaps the food departments of our lives. In the past, we did only what was easy (drive-thru, for example), paying no attention to what really feeds us and our families well. We felt the need only to "fill the hole of hunger" and not nurture and nourish the souls of the humans living in our home—including ourselves.

We have all noticed the paralyzing effects of perfectionism in our lives; this is how our home has become out of control, with CHAOS ruling the roost. Happily, we are coming to terms with perfectionism through our Baby-Steps and routines.

What happens when we hold on to resentment, bitterness, and anger? Perfectionism doesn't allow us to give it up because we want to fix whatever caused it in the first place. How wise is that? Can it really and truly be fixed, or is there a point when you leave it on the altar, so to speak, and release it to God? If you are truly taking BabySteps and cleaning up after yourself, both literally and figuratively, even this type of clutter can be cleaned up, but sometimes someone else has to do some of the picking up. You can control only some things and do what you are able to do; you cannot do it all for someone else. So wringing your hands over what is completely beyond your realm to fix is perfectionism, and this perfectionism is robbing you of precious time that could be invested in someone or something else. We all have the same amount of time in each day: twenty-four hours. Life is too short for obsessing about things we have no control over!

Another area of perfectionism that seems to trap us is being all things to all people. Women are notorious for giving too much and then turning around and being resentful for something they did freely. Now look at that sentence: Whose fault is it? Being angry and indignant when people take the cards you placed on the table in the first place is just plain crazy. There are times when we need to think more like a man. Men can be infinitely more logical than women a lot of the time because they don't conduct life the way we do (although this is a generalization, so just keep reading).

When we are available to everyone for any purpose, we set ourselves up to be taken for granted by everyone: the men in our lives, the children in our lives, and even our friends. People at church or your child's school call you (even when they know you are already over-committed and crazy-busy) because they know you will take on another project you really shouldn't. Why? Because you give too much! And why do you do that? Because in your perfectionism, you want everyone to know how good you are, how perfect you are, and how you are willing to do anything, and I mean *anything*, for the people in your life.

The cost of living such a life? *Staggering!* You have no boundaries and, therefore, you have branded yourself a doormat for everyone to wipe their feet on. The priorities in your life—you and your family—are all left to fend for themselves. You act like a martyr because someone in your house has the audacity to want clean underwear. The kids watch too much TV and don't get their homework done because you're on the phone all night doing for others. You and your family eat a lot of fast food because there is no time to shop for quality food to make a nutritious meal for yourself and for your family.

You are disconnected, discombobulated, and desperately seeking approval, and you never quite get whatever it is you're seeking. And do you know what? You will *never* get it because it is perfectionism driving this out-of-control car, and there is no such destination as Perfect. In life's economy, it does not exist.

So what do we do to combat this tendency? One word: no. Just say no. No, I can't be the captain of the phone chain; no, I can't pick up and drive that package across town in rush-hour traffic, etc. The word "no" spoken firmly and kindly is a powerhouse. Use it frequently! Develop your routines and stick with them. Morning and night you will free yourself from this propensity toward perfectionism and martyrdom. You will make room for yourself and for your family! You will see the freedom in having a schedule that is designed by *you* and not by everyone around you. The junk will fall to the side and a quality life will start to become apparent.

The best part? You will begin to FLY! The effects of FLYing are astounding, and if you take this seriously, you will find yourself writing a very purple, puddly testimonial to FlyLady telling her how truly wonderful letting go is.

So what are you waiting for? Let go of this debilitating perfectionism and FLY with all your heart! Say NO to being everything to everyone and say YES to Baby-Steps, routines, and boundaries. Your life will never be the same!

There is an enormous underlying principle at work here, and that is the fact that each person reading this book right now is worthy of being loved and merits exquisite care. Each and every woman is worthy of being comfortable in her own skin, worthy of giving herself tender, loving care, and worthy of treating her own body like the treasure it is.

We love to complain about our stretch marks, zits, spider veins, and other imperfections that seem to relentlessly grace our body. The older we get, the more plentiful the imperfections. I am guilty of reciting my long list of complaints, too. However, I am starting to realize that with every step and every breath I take, my life is a gift and my body is the "transportation" for my life here on earth. This body is what also houses my soul.

It is worth everything I've got to give the best care to the only body I will ever have. I'm not talking plastic surgery, makeovers, and that kind of thing. I'm talking about the basics: reducing stress, living a life of gratitude, eating well, and moving. I am worth more than nutritionally negative food; a sluggish, sedentary life; and holding on to resentment, anger, and grudges that result in a cold, bitter heart. I am worthy of loving self-care and so are you.

So in that same spirit of worthiness, here are 11 things to help you take care of every inch of yourself. You deserve the best:

1. Understanding that your life is a gift; the care you give your body is how you show thankfulness for that gift.

2.  Recognizing that you are a child of God. You are precious in His sight.

3.  Knowing that when you take care of yourself, there is room to take care of others.

4.  Taking care of yourself helps your inside match up with your outside.

5.  Moving increases endorphins, wonderful hormones that help you feel good. A natural high!

6.  One of the joys in eating real food means no more brain cramps trying to figure out what disodium phosphate and other scary additives are and what they are doing to your body.

7.  Eating real food means you will no longer have to remove your children from the ceiling with a spatula. Your children are calmer. (Just how much fruit is in "fruity cereal" anyway and why are "sports drinks" the color of antifreeze and toilet bowl cleaner?)

8.  Moving with music will help you not only burn calories, but help you "shake your groove thing" and show you that you can still move with the best of them! (Turn on some Bee Gees and see what I mean!)

9.  Drinking water is going to give you pretty skin. Sure, more trips to the potty, but definitely prettier skin!

10. Not hitting the drive-thru will mean more money in your pocket. Stash some of that cash and go get a pedicure!

11. Recognizing that you are worthy of tender self-care means you are FLYing!

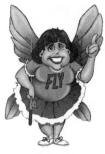

*FlyLady*

We all manage to fool ourselves into believing that this time it will be different! We will stick to the diet, we will work out every day, we will not cheat, our willpower will be strong, and then . . . Well, life happens. One day we wake up and feel that strong urge to take control and just do whatever we have to do to get in shape, get thin, whatever you want to label the frantic thought process we throw ourselves into. We get so carried away in all of our planning that we forget to take time out and really look and see if what we are planning is something that we can actually manage. The first thing that we have to realize is that we are not perfect and we cannot follow any plan or diet "perfectly." If we don't recognize this, we will end up failing and then falling back into our old, unhealthy eating habits and binges along with not moving and, once again, berating ourselves for failing yet again.

First and foremost, we have to remind ourselves that we are worthy of being loved, if only by ourselves. We are worthy of having a happy and healthy body. We deserve to live the best possible life for as long as we are allowed to. There are so many signs that appear that let us know we need to make a change, so why is it that we don't feel that we are capable or give up so quickly?

The problem is our attitude! We are so afraid to start yet another plan because we are afraid we will fail. Or we start a plan with a vengeance and when we can't keep at it, we beat ourselves up over and over again. We tell ourselves that we are just big-boned, or that we are just fine the way we are even if we can't climb more than two flights of stairs. These are some of the excuses we tell ourselves so we don't have to deal with our own Stinking Thinking!

A dear friend of mine had a stroke recently. She is doing well now, but she is no longer living in her own home. One evening we were at book group together and I noticed something about us.

After our book discussion we were offered dessert and coffee. My friend gracefully declined while everyone else was getting a piece of cherry pie and ice cream. When I was offered a piece of pie, I declined, too. I told our host that I was going to be good like Jenny. We had had a lovely dinner three hours earlier and I had not snacked on nuts and grapes during the discussion. I did not feel deprived at all, and I figured out why during the night when the midnight editor visited my sleep.

I was doing it to help my friend not feel so alone. Now I am in great big purple puddles just thinking about it—I could do it for her, but when I am alone I have a problem doing it for me. Why is it so hard for us to be good to ourselves?

Then I thought about being bad and being good. I am not a bad girl; I just treat myself badly by not moving and not putting good food into my body. My friend has had a couple of months of having people teach her a new attitude: that she is worth it—worth eating properly and taking good care of herself.

This story about Jenny was very painful for me because there is stroke history in my family. My mother died from complications of a stroke and arthritis. She was only sixty-five when she died. I watched my mother my whole life as she tortured her body with yo-yo dieting and surgery to get rid of the flab when she would lose the weight, only to gain it all back. Her excess weight played havoc with her knees and hips, making the arthritis worse. I refuse to go through that. My mother was a very unhappy woman and she defined who she was by how she looked on the outside. When she had become bedridden from the trauma to her body, she would tell me that she hoped I, too, would suffer one day as she did so that I would know how much pain she was in. She was so unhappy with herself that she had become the kind of person who would wish that pain and trauma on her own child. She was never able to find happiness and self-worth by loving who she was, only by what she looked like.

Why did I think I was different and special? Why was I fooling myself that I was exempt from the same health issues that have been in my family for years? Well, I am not! My joints have the same problem as anyone who carries around one-hundred pounds of Body Clutter. As I was watching TV one day, I saw a clip from Oprah after she had lost a lot of weight. She wheeled the fat on stage in a little red wagon. When she tried to pick up sixty-seven pounds of animal fat, she could not do it. I used to lug around one-hundred pounds of Body Clutter every day with my legs. I was like a body builder, but the difference was that a body builder gets to put the weights down and my Body Clutter stayed with me all the time. No wonder I used to get so exhausted.

I hate wake-up calls—you know, the ones you ask for in a hotel. I am not even fond of alarm clocks. They wake you up from a zombie state and startle you into awareness. They sound the alarm to get up and get moving. You know that uneasy feeling when your insides are jumpy and you have to get yourself into gear?

When I was forty-eight years and eleven months old I got my very first health wake-up call! It was not one of those gentle little taps on a shoulder, "Honey, wake up." It was a powerful pain in my chest and it scared the living daylights out of me. It started as an uncomfortable feeling after bowling on Friday night. The next day it just hung around and continued to become increasingly more uncomfortable. I had told Robert about the uneasiness and he told me if it got worse to tell him. On Saturday night we were watching a movie with Kelly and Tom and the pain became almost unbearable. I changed chairs in hopes that I was just sitting in a weird position on the couch. Finally at about 11 P.M. I told my family that I needed to go to the hospital. At that point I was scared to death and not thinking straight. They were going to bring Robert's car around to the basement so I didn't have to climb a flight of stairs. I didn't know if I could at that point. Tom helped me stand up and then he sat me back down and instructed Kelly to call an ambulance. In just a couple of minutes the wonderful first responders were there. They checked my blood pressure and pulse. Then the paramedics arrived. They gave me a spray of nitroglycerin under my tongue and put me on a gurney and wheeled me out the door into a waiting ambulance. The pain was not stopping. They started an IV while I was being driven to the emergency room.

When I arrived at the ER, my sweetie was already there and Kelly and Tom were close behind. I have never been afraid of death. In fact, I have discussed these things with my family and the FlyCrew in the event that they have to go on without me. We have discussed this topic with each and every member of our team, but when you are faced with the uncertainty of a chest pain that will not quit hurting, you automatically think the worst. At one point I looked at my sweet darling and could see the terror on his face, even though he was trying to hide it as much as possible from me. He told me I was not going to leave him.

I was trying hard not to cry but the pain at times was almost unbearable. Eventually the doctors concluded that I was not having a heart attack. They said it was pleurisy, which was a bacterial infection in my chest but not in my lungs. After a shot of an anti-inflammatory medication, the pain almost immediately subsided. They gave me some pain medicine to take home with me, and by 2 A.M. I was on my way home—problem solved. Yeah, right!

The next day was Sunday and we were supposed to go to a holiday open house at a dear friend's home. I got all dressed up for the festive occasion and by 3 P.M. I was hurting again and Robert took me back to the ER. I didn't think I could wait for an ambulance. If I thought the pain was bad on Saturday night, it was now over ten on a scale of one to ten! I mean to tell you it was the longest ride I have ever had in his little car. There was no comfortable position I could get in.

Then when I got to the ER, they had trouble getting an IV started. They did all the same tests again. Still I was not having a heart attack, thank the Lord. They must have done more tests, because it seems like I suffered with this chest pain much longer than I had the night before. Even though deep down inside I knew it was not a heart attack, it didn't change the fear you feel when your chest is telling you something else. At one point I felt like I was going to pass out because the pain was so bad. Eventually they gave me the anti-inflammatory shot and I got easy again.

So you see my wake-up call was, in a sense, a false alarm, but one that needed to be heeded! I had the blessing of feeling like I was having a heart attack only to find out that it was not. I know that feeling as though I had a heart attack was a blessing sounds strange, but for me it truly was. I am not sure that I would have really taken my health seriously had I not gone through that experience. My wake-up call was a God Breeze to make me find out what was really wrong with me and what caused the chest pain in the first place.

My dear friend Leanne got me a doctor's appointment

with a friend of hers in Charlotte, and Kelly put me on a plane to see him on Monday. After a number of blood tests, it was confirmed that I had a bacterial infection and I was put on some major antibiotics. They also found that I was anemic and had some sleep problems. I am working on BabySteps to keep me from repeating my family history. My father died of a heart attack at age fifty-eight and my mother of a stroke at age sixty-five. After my wake-up call, I am determined take care of me.

One time when FlyLady was just beginning, Kelly was afraid of getting on an airplane; I remember taking her by the shoulders and saying, "Kelly, God has lots of plans for us. He is not going to allow anything to happen to you!" Then I threw my arms around her for a great big hug and put her on the plane back to Baltimore.

In some strange way, I think God did the same thing with me! He wanted me to know what it is like to suffer a "heart attack" without having permanent damage so that I could see how my life affects so many others. It is a wonderful life; I want to live it and be the healthiest I can be so that my life can continue with those plans that God has for me. I have a choice! I can choose to live well by taking care of me with the tools that God has provided. They are my dear friends who love me and you because I teach best by my example. I want to do this for you and also for me—I want to see my grandchildren grow up and to live a long, happy, healthy life with my sweet darling.

Yes, I had a rude awakening, but when you are walking around not making the right choices, someone has to snap you to your senses. Thank you, God, for opening my eyes, even though it was quite painful at the time. I have many BabySteps to take to keep my health on the right path.

Why was I waiting for that awful wake-up call to encourage me to be kind to myself? I have the family genetics that are warning signals. Now I am choosing to be good to me! I can bless my body by releasing a little clutter at a time. I deserve to live a healthy life—and so do you! Our rebellion only hurts us. This is why I am crying my eyes out on the treadmill as I write this! I have a lot to accomplish with my life and I intend to live it to the fullest!

This next level of FLYing gets us thinking about our reasons for living and loving ourselves on a higher level. I need a home that is comforting to me! We all do. That home is our body! I just want to feel good in my skin!

In order to do that, I have to let go of the Stinking Thinking that has kept me from truly blessing not just myself but also the lives of those who love me and want me to be around on this earth as long as I am allowed to be. I know that I am worth taking care of and worth blessing my heart and body with movement and healthy nourishment. We all have to give ourselves permission to toss that old way of thinking out the door and take BabySteps toward Finally Loving Yourself!

Our journey starts the day we are born and it ends

when we die. Every day we have is a step along our path in life. Some days we may get a little Sidetracked, but for the most part we have learned to stay with our eyes focused on what needs to be done.

When Leanne and I started the Body Clutter phase of our journey, we never dreamed that looking at our own Body Clutter could be such an eye-opening experience for us and that we could translate that experience to help you.

When we first started writing, we were still trapped in our own Body Clutter and Stinking Thinking. With each essay we uncovered another layer of our own perfection. We are Sidetracked by nature and we tend to get burned out real quickly when things don't go as fast as we think they should.

Isn't that what happens when we decide, for whatever reason, that we need to lose weight? We go gung-ho for a time, and then our focus changes and we give up on our quest. Leanne and I were getting frustrated with our journey. We wanted our book finished, but we had lost our drive to complete what we had started.

We could talk the talk, but it wasn't until we started to walk the walk that we found a renewed enthusiasm for our work. In all my years of being saddled with excess Body Clutter, I had never successfully lost any amount of weight. I had fooled myself into believing that I was just fine the way I was. The truth is hard to take when it hits you square between the eyes. I had not really been FLYing!

It was only after I was faced with my own mortality that I made a confirmed decision to change my way of living, not just to take a detour for a few months in order to lose a few pounds. I had chosen to make a real change in my lifestyle. This was my new path, and in order to live I had to follow this path to stay healthy.

I am very blessed because my own reality check was not life threatening even though I thought I was going to die. This is one thing that I hope and pray never has to happen to you in order to get your attention that something is wrong. I do not intend to beat myself up because I had duped myself into believing that I was loving myself. Loving yourself is more than mere words.

"Love" is a verb, an action word, as we learned in third grade. Just saying the word does not make it so. We have to practice the action in order to feel the love that we have for ourselves. We have taken our little acronym FLY to a new level. Finally Loving Yourself is not just something that we say—it is an action that we do. We have to practice it in every aspect of our journey.

When we are not walking the walk and only talking the talk, we are living a lie. This falsehood takes us down a dangerous road of hidden pitfalls and stumbling blocks. We can change our path and head back in the direction of health if we will just do something loving instead of fooling ourselves into believing our own lies.

We have taught you to take BabySteps all along the way, use your timer and, most of all, make your journey fun. When we do some of these simple things, they are acts of love. If that is all that we leave you with, then we have succeeded in getting our message and actions of love across to you.

Are you loving yourself when you skip your daily exercise? I know how we despise the e-word, but when we change it around and call it loving movement, it adds a whole new meaning to the word "exercise." It becomes an action that we do to show ourselves the love that we deserve.

Are you loving yourself when you overeat to the point of feeling stuffed? The guilt that we then suffer is a form of punishment. Why not use an opportunity to eat all you want as a moment for celebration because, instead of acting like a hog that was starving, you stopped yourself and savored every bite?

Are you loving yourself when you push yourself till you are exhausted without taking any breaks? You can learn to pace yourself and not set yourself up for crash and burn.

Are you loving yourself when you go all day without fueling your body? Why not take the time to bless your body with good nutritious food instead of skipping meals and causing your body to go into starvation mode?

Are you loving yourself when you say ugly words to you in your mind or sometimes out loud? We would not speak to our babies that way and it is time to stop this unloving behavior toward ourselves and change those unkind words to words of love and affection.

Everything we do can be an act of love or an act of hate—it is up to you to choose the path. Love your body by taking care of you and you will find that by your actions you are Finally Loving Yourself. Love your body, love yourself.

## Body Clutter Mission

Your Body Clutter Control Journal is waiting for you to write about your attitudes. Just write. Be honest with yourself and don't allow your perfectionism to stop you from eliminating this Body Clutter.

What are the priorities in your life?

Are you a "yes" person?

Have you had any wake-up calls in your life? What were they and how have you reacted to them?

# 11. Your Bathroom—The Scale and the Plumbing

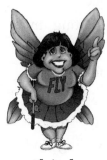

*FlyLady*

When did we begin our love/hate relationship with our bathroom scale? In high school I never really thought about my weight. I ate whatever I wanted because I was active in the marching band and was always on the go. It wasn't until I got pregnant that the scale and the number that it screamed at me became the barometer for my feelings, my dance instructor and diet coach. I want to change the hate relationship with the scale to one of love. We can do this just by removing a little Body Clutter from our brain.

My hate relationship with my scale started during my pregnancy. I refused to look at the scale when I was forced to weigh in at the doctor's office. I will never forget that glorious day I discovered I was eating for two! I had a new license to consume anything I wanted. All I had to do was figure out what that was. So after something sweet, I would have to eat something salty because that just didn't quite fill the craving. Then I went back to the doctor for my monthly checkup. What was the first thing the lovely nurse did? She put me on a great big scale! Then she wrote down that number. Now, as a first time patient I had no clue what to expect from the doctor. I got the whole you-are-not-eating-for-two speech and was told I should gain only twenty-five pounds during my pregnancy. The scale said I had already gained fifteen pounds. So what was I supposed to do? I still had four months to go.

So to keep from being scolded again I learned to play games with my doctor and myself. It started by setting my doctor's appointments late in the morning and skipping breakfast. As soon as I was finished there, I could go pig out. I had a whole month before I had to face that scale again.

During my next visit I complained about swelling fingers, ankles, and feet. I had no clue there was a pill for that. This was my first experience with a diuretic. I could lose five pounds in one day! It is a scary thought now, but my scale said I was happy and doing well—regardless of the fact that I was dizzy and very weak.

Then I was faced with the problem of constipation. I was eating for two, but my "plumbing" was unable to keep up with my constant input of junk! I forgot the most important rule: Eat more fiber. Wasn't there fiber in ice cream and cookies? Hey, there was a pill for this condition, too—

a laxative. That one kept me close to home. My stomach would start rolling and then there would be an explosive reaction to those pills; all of a sudden my plumbing was cleaned out. It is amazing what those scales said after I flushed that toilet!

Here I was allowing the scales to set the tone for my body. I had spent about five months doing the diet dance of torture on the scales at the doctor's office. That is when I developed my hate relationship with my scale. After the baby came I had new destructive tools to help me fool myself into thinking that I was not as big as those scales said I was. This was my mental Body Clutter—the lies I told myself. As I continued to use my Stinking Thinking to help me lose the baby fat, I didn't understand why I just kept gaining; this vicious cycle began my downward spiral of losing and gaining back even more.

When our strong hatred for our own bathroom scale pushes us over the edge, we try a group-effort approach by joining weekly weigh-ins to keep us on our self-destructive path of using diuretics and laxatives. Why not let the groups shame us into doing really strange dances on the scale to help us meet our goal and keep our honor? The sad part is that every dance we do takes us farther away from our elusive goal of peace with our scale. We have tried them all: the diuretic dance, laxative boogie, binge-and-purge polka, and then when all else fails we try the flamingo ballet pose to trick gravity. Why do we allow our self-esteem to be hijacked by a simple machine that gives us a number? We become addicted to those pills to help us make the scale say what we want it to. Then it becomes hard to get off that merry-go-round. Our body can no longer function the way it is designed to because of its dependency on those pills that stop us from eating and help us get rid of water weight and that bloated feeling. It takes BabySteps to help your body adjust to not using the pills. You can do this by drinking your water and eating more fiber—a few raw almonds with a glass of water in the morning and in the evening keep things moving right along, if you know what I mean.

In my quest to reduce clutter, and I mean all types of clutter—physical, mental, financial, and personal—I have been willing to ask some hard questions of myself. This willingness helped me find peace in my life, but I have one more layer of clutter that I need to release—my Body Clutter. So why do I rebel against using a simple tool? What has my scale ever done to me?

I have had to embrace my scale as just another tool with a number to help me see where I am on my journey to better health. I want to look realistically at how I have felt about my scale and why I needed to change my attitude. I have learned many things from my husband, but in my rebellion against the scale, I refused to look at his Morning Routine. My sweetie checks his weight each morning. When I weighed myself, the number that the scale relayed to me caused me to get that sick feeling that I was losing control. I would beat myself up, and then I just threw the baby out with the bathwater. I got rid of a doctor's office scale that my sweet darling used every day. I have come to realize that this number is not a reflection of who I am. It is just a number. Maybe I was suffering from sticker shock. That could be because I have stuck my head in the sand for way too many years. I am determined to get used to seeing the number for what it really is. It is not who I am; it is just what I weigh. I have even gotten used to saying the number out loud and not hiding from it. We now have a new digital scale to help us both with our Morning Routines.

Knowing what I weigh is just like keeping up with a checkbook balance. When you balance that checkbook for the first time in many years, you realize that your fear had created an anxiety that made you avoid it. We cannot allow fear to guide our actions. We have to face our fears head on and with a new understanding. Our scale is just a tool to keep us focused on our BabySteps toward a new way of living.

So as I am getting rid of the sticker shock, I am getting on the scale every day as part of my Morning Routine. This action is not a moment of celebration or defeat. It is the way of starting my day with a focus on my new routine. In fact I have piggybacked this new habit onto other habits that I established several years ago.

My sweetie has been doing this for years. He can see trends in his weight, and as he starts edging up, as we all do from time to time, he uses this information to make good choices about food and movement. Since I have been sticking my head in the sand for many years, I have allowed my weight to creep up and cling to my thighs. This Body Clutter is always with me; I had become immune to seeing it because I had refused to look at my scale.

I want to live a long and healthy life! I have made friends with my scale for the first time ever by seeing it for what it really is—a tool to keep me focused on establishing a new habit.

## Building New Habits: Taking Control

Making friends with our scale is difficult at best. I know I am tempted just to toss it out the window when it does not give me the results that I think I deserve. This is where we have to change our attitude toward this simple little tool. It can give you only information that you put on it. It cannot tell you what you ate yesterday that caused the number to jump up two pounds.

It is up to us to look at the other things we are doing to see what factors are influencing that number between our two big toes. So how in the world can we do it? We have to pretend to be investigators who are trying to unravel this mystery.

Do you remember when we were in third grade and we learned how to do experiments? We set them up and then charted the results. We did them several times to check the outcomes. It was fun. Nowadays on television we see crime scene investigators do this several times a week. We can do it on ourselves.

A woman's weight is never stable. We go through our monthly cycles. One day we feel bloated, the next day our skin is all wrinkled. This morning I got up and weighed my-self. Needless to say I was shocked to see I was up a pound and a half. So I pulled out my Body Clutter Control Journal. It is just a little notebook that I write in to keep up with the things I am doing each day to bless my body.

The first thing I noticed was I had not done any moving yesterday: no walking, no aerobic activity, no weights, and no stretching. But that was not all I had failed to do. I had missed a full meal and two snacks. I didn't take my vita-mins till dinnertime, and I had only one fruit and two veg-etables. Now here is the kicker. I did not cook—we went out to a Chinese buffet. I had written down what I ate, so now I am looking at it. I had a salad with lots of raw vegetables and a little honey mustard dressing on the side. I had four croutons and one egg in the salad.

Overall, it was a meal in itself. But I did not stop at the salad. I went back to get four pieces of sushi and some seaweed salad. I can't have sushi unless I dip it in soy sauce with wasabi dissolved in it. Then I had three chicken wings: barbeque, teriyaki, and spicy hot. I also ate a crab-meat casserole that was drowning in cheese, cream, and butter. In my defense, I had only about one-third of my usual portion. Add to this a serving of stir-fried green beans. For dessert I didn't have cake or cookies (except for the fortune cookie), so I had an egg roll dipped in sweet-and-sour sauce. Oh, and the egg roll and chicken wings were fried.

Having written down what I ate kept me from being mad at my scale. It is not the poor scale's fault that I made bad choices while eating out. I can see from my Body Clutter Control Journal that it is up to me to pick items that are good for me, eat during the day, and make sure I move. All of this fits together in explaining why I was up a pound and a half this morning. The more I use my Body Clutter Control Journal, the easier it will be for me to make good choices when I eat out and when I cook. It may also inspire me to cook more instead of taking the easy path to a restaurant. When I can see on paper the reason that the scale jumped up, it becomes an alarm that gets my attention.

At least at home I know what I have put in our food and how I prepared it. It is so hard to guess when you are eating out. Am I playing Russian roulette with my life when I save up by not eating well during the day and then go to a buffet and pig out? Now here is a really weird part of this little investigation. I thought I was making good choices last night. Maybe the best choice I can make is to stay home, but it is not always a choice that I can make. So I have to use my Body Clutter Control Journal to teach me how to make good choices so I won't blame my scale.

I know there are good choices that I can make at my favorite restaurant. One could be to have them prepare a stir-fry for me. They also have a grill where they will cook the meat I choose. I could leave off the soy sauce and all the fried foods, too. I will continue to keep up with what I eat in my Body Clutter Control Journal and see if the next time I can make better choices and get a different result.

Sometimes we just have to make a game out of the mundane, difficult things in life so we can see if what we are doing is working and make a change if those things are not. Don't blame the messenger when you are the one who made the bad choice. The poor thing is just trying to help you get back on track.

Procrastination is the mother of all guilt. Did you know that? If you're feeling guilty about something, see if that guilt isn't the result of something you've put off doing that you know needs doing. We all do that from time to time, but when it becomes a lifestyle, we lose the joy of living. It doesn't have to be that way.

*Leanne*

But what about constipation? What? That's probably what you just thought when you saw that word. What on earth is she talking about? Have you ever thought of constipation as being your body's way of procrastinating? Really. Think about this for a minute.

When we procrastinate, we're not taking care of things that need to be done. They've been put on the back burner. Yet we know that the nagging feeling that procrastination brings is disrupting our peace of mind and taking away from the fullness of life.

That's exactly what constipation is, too. I know we don't talk about it much, but it's time. If you've ever been there, you know exactly what I'm talking about. It's miserable and while you may not spend your entire life with THAT particular focus, just like procrastination, there's a nagging feeling that haunts you because you need to take care of this problem.

This is an important topic. The majority of pregnant women are constipated at some point during their pregnancy. I remember that well! But nonpregnant women also struggle with this problem and it's no fun. So whether you're currently dealing with this issue or not, read these important tips to get you moving in the right direction, if you catch my drift.

First, you need fiber. There is no fiber in white rice, white flour, or white bread. Eliminate these white things and replace them with brown things: brown rice, whole wheat flour, and whole wheat bread. This will pay off in huge dividends—you cannot afford to eat the white stuff. It's like pouring white glue into your intestines—everything gets stuck. Not only are you not getting the nutrients you need from your food, but you're also slowing digestion way down and setting yourself up for constipation and other fun stuff.

Start reading the fiber counts of the foods you buy and be aware that you need 25 grams of fiber a *day*! Most Americans are lacking in their daily requirement for adequate fiber and the result is a sluggish system that performs poorly.

You can also greatly increase your intake of fiber by eating a ton of veggies. I try to squeeze in two or sometimes *three* with dinner. Chances are good I won't have veggies for breakfast, I may have some lettuce in a salad for lunch, but by dinnertime, I'll really need some veggies. I try to balance my menus with a dark green leafy or cruciferous vegetable (like broccoli) and maybe even a salad, too (not made with iceberg, which is a nearly worthless vegetable). On most days, I try to get in an orange vegetable, too—sweet pota-toes are one of my favorites (and lower in carbs than a white potato by more than half and full of fiber).

Boosting the intake of fiber in one's diet should be tops on the list of anyone hoping to improve her nutritional pro-file and will absolutely keep you on a regular, first name basis with a certain porcelain object in your bathroom, if you know what I mean.

Fiber is much more than your basic oat bran or whole wheat bread. There are two types of fiber: soluble and insoluble. Very easily defined, one is soluble in water and the other is not. And in order to function optimally, we absolutely need both.

Most Americans get only 7 to 8 grams of fiber a day in their diets. But the National Cancer Institute recommends 20–35 grams of fiber daily—a big difference. So then, how do you get the fiber in?

## The Top Eleven Fiber Foods

A starting place to get you going (and for some of you, that may mean literally). Don't forget the water!

1. Beans, Beans, the Musical Fruit. These nutritional wunderkinds are overflowing with fiber. One cup of black beans has over 19 grams of fiber. Worried about the "soundtrack" that comes with them? Try a little bit of ginger in your beans—for some, this turns off the music fast.
2. Bran New for You. Bran cereal is fine, but bran muffins are better! You can get 4 grams of fiber in the average bran muffin.
3. Peas on Earth. Just a half cup will help fill out your fiber quota with over 9 grams of fiber.

4. It's the Corniest. When corn is in season, at 5 grams of fiber per ear, why not eat two ears and get half your fiber for the day? Watch out for too much butter. Don't defeat the fiber value with all the fat!

5. Berry, Berry Good. A cup of strawberries will get you about 3 grams of fiber, but a mere half cup of raspberries has over 4 grams per serving.

6. An Eye for an Eye. Sweet potatoes are pretty potent in the fiber department—5 grams per medium baked sweet potato.

7. Give a Fig. Figs and other dried fruits rate high in fiber attributes—three dried figs equal 10½ grams of fiber while the ol' standby, prunes, clock in at only about 2 grams of fiber for the same amount of fruit.

8. Broccoli Bites. Three-quarters of a cup of cooked broccoli has 7 grams of fiber. Good old broccoli. Is there nothing it can't do? If it could iron, it'd be the perfect spouse.

9. You Really Oater. That stick-to-your-ribs porridge your mom made you on winter mornings has over 7 grams of fiber in a nice, big ¾-cup serving.

10. An Apple a Day. One medium apple has 4 grams of fiber in the form of pectin. It's important to get a wide assortment of fiber in your diet and apples are one of the best.

11. Almond Joy. Just a handful of almonds makes all the difference in the world. Get them raw, keep them in a jar (in the fridge, makes them crunchier), and take a handful twice a day. Watch what happens. Keep drinking your water and you won't believe the results. I've personally seen this—so has FlyLady!

## Turn on the Tap

Fiber is only one part of the equation, though. Start to think about plumbing for a minute. If your garbage disposal is full, the first thing you do before running the thing is turn on the water. Why? It needs the water to get the stuff moving! Notice I said water. I didn't say a can of soda or a cup of tea or coffee. *Water.* Drink it! FlyLady sends out water reminders every day. Sometimes I'm talking on the phone with her and I hear one of her timers go off (she uses several during the day), and that will tell her it's time to hydrate.

I cannot emphasize how important this is. You *need* water. How much? Check your urine—if it is yellow and not clear or nearly clear, you're not getting enough water. Keep drinking and your own body will tell you what you need.

The number one cause of cancer death for women is not breast cancer—it's colon cancer. For the most part, you can prevent this awful disease by being a defensive fiber eater and making sure that your "plumbing" is working. You can do this!

You have heard the expression, "Garbage in/garbage out." Computer techies use this terminology all the time when they refer to the integrity of an operating system. If you care about the integrity of your operating system, take care of it by making sure all things are running smoothly. This is one way to put an end to the ultimate procrastination—constipation.

## Body Clutter Mission

It is time to get out your Body Clutter Control Journal again. (Don't you love that you are not being graded on this?) Remember, these Body Clutter Missions free you from your perfectionism.

Write down how you feel when you get on a scale. Just get it out. When did you start to feel this way?

Look at your scale as a tool. Use it every day to see if what you are doing to release your Body Clutter is working or if you need to change the amount of fiber in your diet, water consumed, or your moving.

# 12. Plateaus

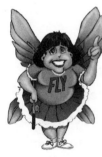

*FlyLady*

Until recently I had never really successfully lost any weight in my life. The truth is that I was scared to try because I didn't want to fail. Now that I have made the decision to take care of myself by eating better and moving more, I have started to see a daily change in the number that is my body weight. That number has become a barometer for me to use each day. It is not a guide for how I am going to berate myself. I have quit beating myself up over that number between my feet.

Since making the decision to take control of my Body Clutter, I have started to lose weight. It has been a slow and steady process. Right now I want us to look at what happens in our mind when that number between our feet gets stuck and quits going down. This is a plateau. You have heard many people talk about those last few pounds being the hardest. Well, my plateau hit at a loss of thirty-five pounds. The first pounds seemed to be falling right off me. I am still in shock that I am in a new size. I continue to reach for those perfect size twenty-twos. Right now that size swallows me whole. One minute I am celebrating and the next minute I am crying. So what is all of this emotion about?

Part of the emotion comes from having actually lost any weight at all! This is strange new territory and I have not ventured into this area before. I guess there is a lot of fear associated with this initial surge of emotion. What are we afraid of? Is it losing the weight? I think the fear has to do with gaining it back. We have all seen this happen to friends when they have lost some weight.

But I want to address the plateaus that will occur in the journey toward a healthier life. Plateaus are just a way for our body to tell us that our metabolism has gotten used to what we are doing and it is time to tweak our routines just a little. Many times the plateau can be celebrated because you did not re-collect Body Clutter during a holiday or vacation. It is all in how we look at it. But we have to look! We can't just keep our head in the sand and speculate about what is happening to our body. This is why weighing ourselves on a daily basis gives us the tools to know when our metabolism has gotten bored with our new lifestyle.

There could be another reason that we don't seem to be losing any more of our Body Clutter. We may have stopped what we were doing and returned to our old ineffective habits. That is why charting your daily activity, how many times a day you are eating, and what you are eating is going to help you better assess what is going on with your body. I can usually tell when I have quit eating three meals and three snacks. I can also recognize when I am not drinking my water and eating too much sodium and not enough fiber. This is not represented by a constant weight but by a little weight gain. I don't beat myself up over the day-to-day gain or loss; I look at what I did the day before to help me understand the simple number.

When I look at the overall numbers from one month to the next, this is when I can see the plateau. Again, I don't beat myself up. I reinforce the habits that I have been doing. I celebrate that I have not added Body Clutter and keep taking BabySteps toward a healthier lifestyle.

It is when I find that my routines have not fallen by the wayside that I begin to tweak my habits by adding another one to the ones I have successfully established. My new plateau is evidence that it is time to step up my moving routines. I have added some weight training to my basic weekly plan. Another thing I can do is add some moving to my afternoon or evening. So instead of once a day, I am moving in the mornings *and* evenings. But you won't be able to see this if you are not keeping up with it in your Body Clutter Control Journal.

Now I know this may sound strange, but another reason for a plateau is that I may not be eating enough, and this alone tells my body that I am in starvation mode. I may have to put a few more calories into my meals and snacks in order to increase my metabolism. When your body goes into starvation mode, your metabolism slows down. Your body is trying to reserve every calorie for later to protect you from not having enough food. We have to play tricks with our food and our moving to get our metabolism out of starvation mode. That is why eating breakfast is so important for us.

When we refuse to eat breakfast, we are telling our body that we are not going to have any food today. When we finally do eat, our body is going to save those calories for later. Those calories become the Body Clutter on our thighs and backside. If you are not charting your food, water, and exercise, you are not going to be able to see your plateaus or the fact that you are not following your routines. This is all about being honest with yourself.

Keep in the front of your mind that there is no vacation from your new lifestyle. So when you go on a trip, it is important for you to eat like you would at home. You can still make good choices, and those good choices will help you release your Body Clutter. At the same time I don't want you to feel deprived when you go to your favorite restaurant. Practice not eating the whole thing. Share a meal with a friend. You still get to enjoy your special meal. If you start to feel deprived, you have to stop and think about this. What is happening? Have you really made a choice to change, or are you feeling sorry for yourself? Are you allowing yourself to sabotage your new lifestyle? You are not going to recognize these things if you are not willing to address them head-on.

Plateaus can also be the result of coasting till we are ready to take our next step—like taking a staircase to the top of a big building. It goes round and round and all along the way there are landings. At each landing you catch your breath and make the decision to take the next flight of steps. We can't even see the top of the staircase but we know it is there. All we are concerned with is taking the next step. Each BabyStep is a habit in our routine. Putting one foot in front of the other and lifting yourself up becomes automatic, then you hit the landing and you get to rest but it is only for a little while. Don't allow the plateau or landing to keep you from taking your automatic steps.

My sweet darling loves to bake cookies. He is really good at coming up with new recipes. I can have one small bite to sample his latest creation and rave about them. I don't have to eat ten cookies to enjoy my sweetie's cookies. We have to practice our new habits and not fall victim to our old way of thinking. In the past I would have felt deprived; now I celebrate that I can savor one bite and not have to mindlessly eat several to have an opinion.

I want you to think about these plateaus in the same way you think about your house. Just because your routines keep your home in order and your sink shining doesn't mean you can allow your routines to fade away. You keep doing them even though your home looks good. Because when you stop, you will begin to see your clutter come back and your home will end up in CHAOS again. None of us wants to go back there. As your home habits become automatic, your new lifestyle habits will feel good to you, too. Each month you can add a new habit to practice. You are going to have so much to celebrate!

We all are immune to our own clutter. We get complacent with our new lifestyle routines to the point that we don't even realize that we are doing them. We can also be so happy with our results that we feel we deserve a reward. Don't allow yourself to get caught up in your old way of thinking, and you know exactly what I am talking about—"I have been doing so good that I deserve to eat a cookie!"

It takes looking hard at your routines and at yourself to see clearly when you have hit a real plateau. Most of the time what we perceive as plateaus are just momentary lapses in our routines that accumulate. There is a moment for celebration because this plateau or lapse in our routines has not resulted in weight gain and falling back into our old ineffective habits. All we need to do is tweak our routines or get back to our basics.

Celebrate and investigate! Don't beat yourself up. You have the power!

As frustrating as plateaus can be, they can also be a place of respite while you figure out what the heck is going on in your life. I say this from a very personal experience that helped me understand that *everything* counts—food, movement, attitude, and stress.

*Leanne*

A few years ago, my husband and I had just separated and the stress was extraordinary. Just prior to this separation, I had been working out hard with a personal trainer. I was eating right and working out, and yet the weight stubbornly stuck to me. I was losing a little here and there, but it was very, very slow, and plateaus became a way of life. This was the first of a series of little plateaus; the next big one came after a hugely stressful event in my life that required a physician's help. Keep reading . . .

By the time the separation actually came down, my exercise started to dissipate as the worries and cares of all this marital discord came crashing down hard. I lost the desire to create anything healthy in my own kitchen and though I tried desperately to make good decisions eating out, I didn't. That was because my primary concern with food was for comfort, not nutrition. I began to look at food as a means of escape. I had done this before in my life so it wasn't new territory, although the enormous weight gain was.

The result of this so-called comfort? I gained thirty pounds in three months. By the time FlyFest in Chattanooga came, I was wearing very tight size eighteen pants. I really needed a bigger size, but my pride wouldn't let me go shopping for the right size. Instead, I looked for the 1X and 2X tags on clothing so I didn't have to face the truth. In my (minor) defense, I didn't eat that badly, nor had I completely abandoned my exercise program. Things changed, though, and my BabyStep habits had become sporadic. Add to that the most incredible stress I've ever been under in my life, including full-blown panic attacks.

What I learned from this experience is the importance of consistency. Notice the word "consistency," not "perfectionism." Perfectionism demands absolutely no change, no slipups, and no deviation. Perfect is impossible to make happen, while consistent asks only that you keep it up. The difference, too, is that consistent won't beat you up but will encourage you to make up for it the next day, while perfect will tear you down to your underwear and berate you, causing you to throw the whole thing aside and give up.

I also learned that reducing the stress in your life is critical to your health. Stress causes disease and sickness. For example, it blew out my thyroid. That was an additional reason for the thirty-pound weight gain, not just the sporadic nature of my food consumption and irregular movement.

But prior to getting a flat tire on my thyroid, I had been on a disproportionate plateau. I was stuck at two hundred pounds. I was eating right, I was exercising. I was convinced that I needed some kind of radical new diet, that I needed to find the right combination of exercise (weight lifting and aerobics), but couldn't quite get my hands around it. I was also working very hard and, not surprisingly, was burning the candle at both ends. I had a job as a radio talk-show host in Southern California and the burden was mine alone to produce a quality, one-hour call-in talk show, aired live Monday through Friday. I was also writing another book and had the responsibility of a home, kids, and a husband (and I knew that the husband part wouldn't last much longer). The stress was eating me alive and the weight barely budged—and, for the most part, stood still. I was beyond frustrated. I just wanted to get *one thing* under control in my life!

Postseparation, when I had gained as much weight as I had, I was thoroughly bummed out and really hard on myself. I was angry that I had "let myself go." The reality of the situation was that I was two inches away from checking myself in somewhere to keep from falling apart. What kept me together at that time was a terrific doctor (who finally diagnosed my thyroid condition) and unbelievable friends—most notably FlyLady, who walked through this fire with me every step of the way. I will never forget her consistent and calm presence in my life during that time. The incredible part of this whole story is that she was living in North Carolina at the time and I was still in California. We stayed in touch via phone, cell phone, email, and instant message. She held me together and kept me from falling over the edge.

After I came home from FlyFest, I thought it was time to get it together in the weight department of life. "Enough is enough," I said to myself. "This time, I'm going to get serious." Well, that never happened, and although I never gained any more weight, I couldn't lose any either; but then again, my movement and food were inconsistent and the Body Clutter between my ears wasn't helping either. I was still too much of a perfectionist and thought it had to be an all-or-none proposition.

But it was on the plateau of weighing 230 pounds that I finally discovered that who I am and what I will be in my life will never be measured by the size of my jeans or the color of my lipstick, but rather by my character and what kind of person I am. I also realized that holding onto this Body Clutter was an acceptance of the human, fleshy shield that I had built out of fear. I was no longer fearful, therefore, I was no longer in need of that kind of protection; so I used that moment on that flat surface (the plateau) to let go of emotions and feelings that no longer needed to live inside me. It was time to let go and I finally did, but not until I came to that flat place of contemplation—it was the plateau that changed my life and moved me in a brand-new direction.

## Body Clutter Mission

Open your Body Clutter Control Journal and look back at the past month.

If you have not started keeping a Body Clutter Control Journal, then do it *now*. Grab an old three-ring binder and put some paper in it. Each day weigh yourself and write it down. Also write down what you eat, when you eat, how much sleep you are getting, how much moving you are doing, and your water and vitamin intake. Also write down how you feel and what is happening in your life. This will help you when you hit your plateau. We have a page for you to download in our website:

www.FlyLady.net

There are times when our plateaus are not real plateaus, but instances where our routines are falling by the wayside.

Ask yourself these questions to see if you have not been doing your routines.

Have you caught yourself hiding from someone while you eat?

Have you neglected to chart your weight daily?

Have you been drinking your water?

Have you been eating on the run in the car?

Have you been staying up too late?

Are you skipping meals and snacks?

Are you are too busy to shop for groceries?

Are you getting dressed and fixing your face in the morning?

Have you written down what foods you are eating?

Have you refused to eat your vegetables?

Have you been too busy to Bless Your Heart?

# 13. The Anger and Fear . . . and Food

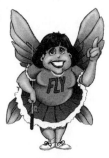

*FlyLady*

After writing everything in these past chapters, there is still more that we have to address. When planning this book we had to ask ourselves, "What is the message that we want to give you?"

We realized that while we want to teach you how to take BabySteps and create routines that will help you deal with your Body Clutter issues, there is more. There are times when we have to take a really hard look at what is going on in our lives beyond the ins and outs of everyday life. There are different circumstances and situations that somehow still keep us from being able to free ourselves enough to take those BabySteps toward getting rid of our Body Clutter.

Earlier in the book we discussed using food as a weapon

of self-destruction. We can take that a step further to discover that we also use food as a defense mechanism when
we feel that we have been hurt or even abused. Abuse
comes in many forms, and its effects can ruin any good intentions we may have about coming to terms with our Body
Clutter. Nowadays the word "abuse" is used, and overused,
in many different ways, but in this case we are referring to
the mental, verbal, emotional, and even physical types of
abuse, past or present. The situations in which we may find
ourselves abused also vary.

Abuse can be found in family relationships, love relationships, friendships, and even in churches and at our
jobs. There are times that we are involved in toxic relationships and we are not even aware of it. We are yelled
at, pushed around, and manipulated. We find ourselves
either lashing back or just taking it because we are not
sure how to break the pattern that keeps bringing us back
into these situations. When in any emotionally abusive
situation, we all find ourselves dealing with two very specific reactions: anger and fear.

Sometimes we find ourselves taking on roles in our
adult lives and we are not even aware of it; we never
even imagined they could exist within us. We often find
ourselves instinctively in these roles when we are faced
with various situations. Let's take a look at some of these
roles:

**The Pleaser:** We want everything to be okay and running
smoothly, so there is never any tension or flared tempers.

**The Ostrich:** No matter how difficult or strained things are, we just bury our head in the sand waiting for things to get better. When circumstances don't get better, we just stick our head in deeper in the hope that everything will disappear.

**The Self-Preservationist:** We take and take whatever is handed out to us because we know it is just easier to swallow it than actually to confront what is happening around us.

**The Protector:** We defend everyone we love and go into Mama Bear mode to make sure that no one will get close enough to hurt our loved ones—or us.

**The Excuser:** We make excuses, not just for others around us but for ourselves as well. We always have an excuse for why something has happened or why something has not happened.

**The Perfectionist:** We always look for everything around us, including the people in our lives, to be perfect in every way, yet perfection is something that neither we nor they are ever able to achieve—a sure setup for failure.

In all of these roles we find ourselves stuck in the same issues: anger and fear. We take that anger and fear and turn them inward against ourselves. If that is not recognized or dealt with when it is happening, we find ourselves back in the same place over and over again—the refrigerator, drive-thru, or grocery store. We are on the fast track to food, trying to soothe our anger and fear, but it is never quite enough.

We need to address how we perpetuate the hurt and pain that we have suffered by turning our anger inward on ourselves and how we can stop this pattern of behavior. This is our Body Clutter. It is not just the thunder thighs or the double chins; it is the accumulation of those hurtful words and actions and the resulting pain that have hard-wired us with the instinctual action to protect ourselves. When we allow ourselves to get too hungry, too angry, too tired, or too lonely, our instincts take over and we lose control of our thought processes as well as our self-control. We are not aware that when we reach for food to comfort us that we will still be left with the pain and the hurt after the last bite, time and time again. As women, we don't ever like to be out of control; for us it is a survival mechanism.

There are reasons behind every action. We may not even know why we react the way we do, but with patience and a willingness to get to the heart of the matter we can grow past those instinctual responses and eventually catch, and even stop, ourselves in the middle of one of our self-destructive patterns. It is this taking hold of our emotions that is going to stop us from perpetuating the abuse. Maybe the next time we feel the old pattern start up, we will be able to recognize those feelings before they explode and cause us to hurt ourselves with food.

## Anger—Red-Hot or Ice-Cold?

When you are in a situation that is causing pain, anger, or fear, what are you feeling inside your body? Sometimes we don't know the signs and they can be different for each of us. Do you feel your face turn red? Do you break out in a rash? Do your ears get hot? Do tears start to well up in your eyes? Do you hold your breath? If you can talk, do your words get louder and louder trying to make the other person hear you? Or are you withering in silence, unable to get a word out? Are you both talking at the same time and no one hears what the other one is saying? You have heard of red-hot anger—here it is.

One way to handle angry feelings is not to immediately react, but instead just to listen intently as if you were an outside person who was trying to figure out the process. We need time to gather our thoughts. It is fine if we can't think of things to say back, because sometimes those responses make things worse. At times like these, all we want is for the person who is abusing us to stop. If you do get a chance or a moment to speak, try asking, "What can I do to help this situation?" A lot of times this simple question brings a calming level to the issue—gentleness is the key. Once the abusive behavior has stopped, there is a good chance that you both can process what just happened. It is never easy facing our fears and taking responsibility for our role in the drama.

Anger is usually the emotion that we keep bottled up inside us. We hold it in and then, from time to time, we allow our bottle to be shaken, only to explode in a rage and then, once again, turn to food for comfort. So how can we constructively deal with anger and not turn it on ourselves? We can pick up a phone and call a friend and say, "Hey, I just need to vent." We can sit down at the computer or with a piece of paper and start to write about what is making us angry. We don't have to let anyone else see it. We just have to get it out! We can take a walk around the block with a favorite furry friend. That pent-up anger is what has caused us to hurt ourselves by overeating, overspending, working too hard, not getting enough rest, not exercising, and lots of other ways we have found to punish ourselves.

We are no longer the whipping post for everyone's anger and fear, including our own. When we can catch ourselves, we can begin to heal. Knowledge is going to save us from ourselves, and these loving tools below are going to help us learn to cope with our anger and fear.

**All You Need Is Love**
Love—there it is, that very word that brings us all back to what is really important. Loving yourself enough to take your first BabySteps on the journey to living a life with peace and hope rather than fear and anger. We all want to feel love and have that love validated by others, yet there are so many times that we are unable to love our-

selves first. Loving yourself is a work in progress; you will never be finished. Love is always something that must be nurtured.

For the first ten years of my life I was my mother's protector. Every time Daddy would get mad and try to hit her, I would try to defend her by standing in front of her. There were times that I was tossed across the room to get me out of the way. I also protected my sisters from our mother. When she was feeling unloved or unattractive we knew it through her episodes of rage and unhappiness. We thought it was bad when Daddy was with us, but it got worse when they divorced.

My mother was never able to love herself enough to understand that she was worthy of being cherished and treated with love. She was able to view her self-worth only by her physical appearance and then validated that self-worth through the attention of men. There were prescription drugs to help her lose weight and keep her happy. There were plastic surgeries to keep her as attractive as she thought she had to be. She never felt she was complete unless she was in a relationship. She looked to others for fulfillment. She was never cognizant of the character of the men she dated—as long as there was a man around to complete who she was as a person, that was good enough.

She was searching for love and was unable to see that some of the men she chose were not safe to have around children. I can speak only for myself, but a few of those men were predators and, as a twelve-year-old, I knew I had to keep them away from my sisters. My hardwiring was installed, and once it was in place it was very diffi-cult to remove.

It all boils down to not feeling worthy of being loved. We set ourselves up for failure because deep down inside we can't believe that we could be someone who is lov-able. Years ago I thought that the deep, dark secret within me was my messy house, but now I see that I was always protecting that little girl inside me from being hurt again—that was really my dirty little secret.

Every living soul wants to feel loved, and somewhere along the line, we convince ourselves that it is our fault if we are not loved in the way we think we should be. We then find ourselves taking abuse and hurt from people in our lives whom we are really craving love from.

I did just that in my first marriage. I suffered mental anguish thanks to a man who was determined to make himself feel better by degrading me. Day after day I was reminded that I was nothing and he was everything be-cause he had a college degree. I also suffered (in silence) with constant insults that I was fat and, guess what? I weighed only 150 pounds. The more he complained, the fatter I got. I would catch myself stuffing my face in front of the refrigerator, devouring anything I could find to keep from confronting him because I was afraid he would stop loving me in any form. After all, I had a home and a son to raise, and I didn't think I could do it alone. So with the hardwiring from my childhood, I protected what I had by taking the insults and stuffing my feelings to keep the rage from exploding.

When the people who claim to love us more than anyone else treat us in ways that are truly unmentionable to others, we go back to what brings us comfort. Food never turns us down, talks back, is mean or unkind. Food never treats us with disrespect or leaves bruises on our heart, mind, or body. Or does it?

The problem with using food to comfort ourselves is that in reality we are continuing the abuse. When we use food to insulate us from the abusive tendencies of others, we are only hurting ourselves and adding to the Body Clutter that we want to get rid of. Do you see the vicious cycle? An example of this is when someone has really hurt our feelings or, worse, physically hurt us. The minute he or she is gone, we turn to the refrigerator to soothe our feelings. As we are spooning that ice cream down our throats, like applying an ice pack to our raw emotions, our minds go into overload, creating conversations in our heads of things that we wished we had said. Instead of taking time to sort out the words and actions, we keep eating and eating, searching for comfort. The problem is that the comfort is only temporary and the irony is that we are not hurting those who hurt us—we are hurting ourselves.

You may not feel that you are able to take control of the abuse you are suffering, but you do have the ability to stop the endless torture of hurting yourself. When you give yourself permission actually to look at what is hurting you and causing you to be fearful, you have peeled back the first layer to loving yourself.

I don't have all the answers or even all the questions, but I do know that we must start with loving ourselves. When we truly love ourselves, we will not put up with abuse any longer. As we remove the layers of clutter in our home, we will also be releasing some of our own Body Clutter. I have warned people many times that if you are in an abusive situation, as your home gets cleaner, the abuse will get worse. I think that happens because abusers feel they are losing control. That loss of control is what they hate most. Usually, they were victims, too. It is very sad that we were hurt as children, but that does not excuse being an abuser of others—or yourself. Yes, you heard me right. You have been abusing yourself because of your lack of love for you! It is up to each of us to stop the abuse right here.

I believe that the only way we can feel worthy of love is to take BabySteps to repair the damage, simple Baby-Steps that teach us to nurture that scared little child that is inside each of us. That little baby just wants to be held, and there is no one in the world who can do that for you but you! No man or woman is ever going to fulfill that desire. It has to come from your own heart. By now we have all heard, You can't love another till you truly love yourself first. Don't write this off as self-centeredness—it is really a selfless act! Once you begin to love yourself, you will find your capacity to truly, selflessly love others! I know you think you are already doing that, but wait and see just how much love you can give when your cup is overflowing because you have taken care of you!

I know you want immediate gratification here, but we might just need to fake it to get started. Fake it till we make it! This is pretty sound advice. So let's figure out ways to make ourselves feel loved.

Here are some ideas that worked for me:

**Be kind to yourself.** Do not completely deprive yourself of things you love. Diets are notorious for self-punishment. You don't have to eat the whole quart of ice cream in order to nurture yourself. Sometimes all it takes is a spoonful.

**Keep food in your home that is good for you.** You can't eat it if it is not in your house. Keep your pantry filled with nutritious snacks and ingredients to fix wonderful, healthy meals.

**Don't starve yourself by skipping meals or saying you don't have time to eat.** Take time to refill your gas tank regularly. It is when we are running on empty that our injured-baby instincts take over and we can't think clearly. We can't even analyze what is happening at the time. You can't think straight on an empty stomach.

**Face your feelings.** When you feel yourself getting antsy, please stop and figure out why that feeling has arisen. I do that by writing as fast and as hard as I can. I call it my "brain dump." Use your Body Clutter Control Journal. Practice writing down your feelings—it's a good way to dissect them and get to the bottom of what is hurting you. If you are afraid someone may find it and read it, you don't have to have a book. You can just type it and then put it in a folder named Recipes. No one will ever look in it.

**Get yourself at least one outfit that you feel like a million bucks in.** Don't ever wear anything that makes you feel frumpy. You are a beautiful person!

**Drink your water.** Dehydration causes you to feel fatigued. Buy yourself a pretty glass to drink it from and drink some water every hour. Use a timer to remind yourself.

**Take a break occasionally.** Try closing your eyes for a few minutes and meditating every hour. Little breaks taken regularly recharge your batteries so you are not stressed out as much. You deserve time for yourself.

**Pamper yourself with your favorite music.** It doesn't matter if anyone else in the house likes it. Get a Walkman or an iPod with earphones. Music is the medicine that flows over you and heals all that hurts.

**Turn off the television, close the newspaper.** For now, quit listening and reading about the bad things that are happening in the world. If you need to know about something, someone will tell you! Fill your heart and soul with good things.

**Listen to inspirational tapes and motivational speakers.** Listen to them over and over again. You have many years of hardwiring you have to reprogram. Eventually you will begin to believe what they are saying.

**Say only nice things to yourself.** When you hear negative words come out of your mouth or you think them, stop right there and change them to a positive message—you can do this. The hardest thing to do is catch yourself in the act. The more you do it, the better you are going to feel. You are breaking the bad habit of abuse. You have heard it from others for so long that you have started doing it to yourself. Stop it now!

**Take bubble baths.** Relaxing in warm water relieves the stress and tension that is in your body. The warm water is a womb that gives birth to a refreshed you. Let the water take all your troubles down the drain.

**Release any guilt that you feel.** Apologize to the people you love and watch the changes that occur in each relationship. The most important thing that you can do is forgive yourself. It doesn't matter if others forgive you or not. This is not their battle. Forgive yourself and that release of guilt will help you to FLY—Finally Love Yourself!

**Forgive others and quit harboring grudges.** Hatred is a pill you take to kill the person who has harmed you. Forgive him or her and get on with living. It may be hard at first. If you have to, concentrate on wishing good things for that person or pray for him or her. You can do this. I promise it won't make you sick. I like to do this when I am in the bathtub. This is another bad feeling that goes down the drain with the old, dirty bathwater.

**Go to bed at a decent hour.** You need your rest—try to get at least eight hours of sleep. Getting enough sleep makes us much happier when we're awake.

**Only have things in your home that make you smile.** You deserve to walk around with happy thoughts in your mind. If you have items in your home that make you feel bad when you look at them, they need to go away.

We abuse ourselves in ways other than overeating. Look for ways to stop all forms of abuse. It is only an action away! We can reverse the years of hardwiring and find our true self for the first time ever. I promise.

Throughout this book, I've shared my own pain about the fleshy shield I formed for myself and why. I've shared my past and my marriage. I've also shared stories about the abuse and my reactions to it and how it helped me build a flesh wall to keep out the pain. What I haven't talked about is the anger—both toward yourself and toward those who have hurt you. In my mind there are different degrees and types of anger, most of it being very unhealthy, but some of it being healthy. You will see what I mean in a minute.

*Leanne*

The biggie of course is rage—an out-and-out violent, out-of-control anger that drives people to do things they regret later. A synonym for rage is insanity. That thought ought to help you steer your boat away from that storm!

Then there is resentment, which is an inner anger that will usually show up in audible sighs or statements of martyrdom—"Well, I guess I'll just have to do it myself [big, heavy sigh]. No one around here will help me." Resentment, when strong enough, will also rear its very unattractive head in fits of rage. You want to deal with resentments, grudges, and other kinfolk to this destructive emotion before they get a foothold in your life.

Indignation and entitlement, I believe, are closely connected and come from a distorted view of the world. Some people get indignant having to wait in lines or being caught in traffic. It's almost as if they feel, for some reason, they shouldn't have to wait. They're above waiting (or whatever it is that they have become indignant over).

People with entitlement issues see themselves, too, as being above situations. An example of this is someone I know who doesn't feel he should have to work for a living and that everyone else should pay his way while he "works" as an artist. The problem is that his "art" doesn't pay his way, and while he's nearly fifty years old, he becomes angry if confronted with this fact.

All of these types of anger (often manifested in the same person's life) are destructive and leave a path of ruin wherever they're allowed to run amok. I'm sure you know people in this situation and perhaps you are a person like this and the anger has all but taken away your life.

Anger plus food, alcohol, or drugs are often fast friends and a destructive duo in lives with out-of-control emotions. Most people with Body Clutter issues understand the food/anger connection and have eaten to stifle emotions, feelings, or hurt.

There is another side to anger—the constructive side. Now understand what I'm saying. *All* of the above types of anger are completely destructive. What I'm talking about is the hidden anger we have inside us, the kind that manifests itself as depression, frustration, and despair. Here's the cool thing, though. Once you understand what that depression, frustration, and despair are all about, once you understand the big picture and can connect the dots, you are halfway there to getting it dealt with—the construction vs. the destruction of *you*. That's the constructive side of anger.

For me, the halfway point came in the form of anger. It wasn't rage, despair, entitlement, or indignation. It was a pure anger. In other words, I finally understood what was going on in my life and that I didn't have to live that way anymore if I chose not to. I had a *choice*, and that was the beginning of my own personal liberation.

Later on, after making a huge decision about my marriage, I discovered the anger. Boy, was I mad! It was a red-hot anger—toward my ex-spouse, toward myself, and toward God. Once I recognized it, I dealt with it. I prayed hard for the words and I finally told my ex that I was angry with him and here were the reasons why. I asked his forgiveness for my failures in the marriage, and then I had a good cry and was done.

I wasn't worried about my anger with God—He was big enough to handle puny, little me. We had quite a few conversations that summer and I cried my eyes out. The cool thing was I finally broke through the why-me-God stuff (I answered myself, "Well, why not me?") and got to the place of seeing God as my Father and climbing up on His adequate lap and allowing His presence to fill my heart. Then the anger dissolved into peace.

The problem child was *me*. I kept bringing up stuff over and over again and then beating myself up. I should have known better. I should have waited. I should have asked my mother. I should have asked Santa Claus for advice. Well, not quite, but you get the drift. Poor Marla had to listen to this junk for an entire summer, and one day she just calmly said to me, "Leanne, you have two beautiful children, your life is on track now, we have a mission from God to accomplish, but you have to stop this." I don't know why, but it clicked that time and I finally let go of all that anger. It was what it was and no more—it was time to move on and live.

This is my prayer for you: that you will see how potent anger is and how it can rob you of your life. It will put on the Body Clutter. It will destroy relationships and totally remove any joy that you could have in your life. Anger has got to go. Read the Mission at the end of this chapter for some solid action you can take. When you lose the anger, you lose the Body Clutter. I know this to be the truth!

## Body Clutter Mission

Your Body Clutter Control Journal is going to help you more right now than ever before. Pour out your heart. Tell your perfectionism to go away! This writing is just for you.

What are you afraid of?

Whose voice do you hear in your head?

What do you want to say to that voice?

Write it now in your Body Clutter Control Journal.

What happens when you do not have the words to say what you feel? Use your Body Clutter Control Journal to get it out of you. The writing will help you figure out what your feelings are.

Now turn any negative words you have heard into positive, comforting words to bless your body. Write them here so you can look at them and know what to say till you have silenced those abusive words. Say them over to yourself out loud. Hear your positive words fill your head—these will replace the abuse.

# 14. If You Don't Do It— Who Will?

Dear Readers,

Closing a book like this is not easy and I want to address you all personally. There is so much to say still, even at the end of the book! As I sat down to write this, I wondered how to send you off and wish you well when I know you're starting the same journey I am still on. I want to encourage you and give you hope, but I also don't want to sell you a bill of goods that says it's fast, it's easy, and it's only $9.95—like some hawker of weight-loss gadgets on late-night TV.

Socrates said that the unexamined life is not worth living. It's the "examining" part that can get sticky. Another man known for his simple observations, Benjamin Franklin, adds the perfect addendum to Socrates' profound statement. "Life is difficult," said Ben. No kidding!

*Leanne*

When I started to get up close and personal with my own Body Clutter, I was amazed at how much "stuff" came up. Emotional, physical, mental, and even spiritual challenges became, and are still, part and parcel of the process. I used to dread having to walk through these types of valleys, but the most important thing I've learned is that this journey, while incomplete, is what makes my life so much more fulfilling and real. Avoiding the pain of such honesty is what made me feel hollow and purposeless. This is big stuff for me.

A while back, I went shopping for clothes at a store for women my size. I didn't buy dowdy, ugly clothes; I bought cute jeans and T-shirts, linen blouses, and a really darling denim jacket I had always wanted. I bought bras that fit and weren't designed for a skinny lingerie model. I splurged and didn't skimp—and I did not allow myself to think that one day I would be back in my size-six jeans and just needed some things "to get by on" for now. The thing is, for the longest time, I used to hate shopping for clothes because I dreaded the dressing room mirror. This time, I had a ball! The big lesson was celebrating who I was right then and there and not waiting. My insides finally connected with my outside and that's when the Body Clutter really started to come off and has stayed off.

There are times in our lives when we don't listen to ourselves. We don't listen to God, either. Instead, we listen to the wrong voice—the one that puts us down and tells us we're nothing unless we're the "right" size. I listened to it for too long. I know the outside me might be a little bigger than it was twenty years ago, but I sure love the inside me a whole lot better. I am a woman who has finally grown up and has seen that it's okay to be herself. It's a liberating thing to love yourself just as you are today and not for what you can be tomorrow. Today is a good place to be.

So what do I want you to come away with now that the end of the book is here? Just what I came away with from writing the book: You are truly worth loving just as you are today. God has a plan, a purpose, and reason for you to be here on this planet and it isn't so you can fit into smaller jeans. We have given you some wonderful ideas in these pages to help you deal with your Body Clutter, but one thing I have to mention again is that you must, *today* stop the self-abuse and the awful, negative self-talk.

You are beautiful and worthy of the most tender, loving care you can lavish on yourself. Look in the mirror and thank God for putting you here. You are His child, and as a daughter of the King, you are to treat yourself royally: good, healthy food for your beautiful body, movement to keep your heart happy, and an attitude that is thankful and positive. This royal treatment will serve you well on your journey and will take you to where you want to go.

There are no limits!

Love,

*Leanne*

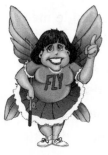

*FlyLady*

Dear Friends,

This book is the wake-up call that we all have been searching for. We have purchased every kind of self-help book that has been written looking for the way to get rid of the feeling that we have to fix what is wrong with us. The truth is that we just need to give ourselves the tools to handle stress when it unconsciously triggers the pain that we have suffered.

We just wish we could hold you and tell you that everything is going to be all right! That may not be physically possible, but know in your heart that we are here and it is our wish for you that the healing start by getting rid of the hardest clutter of all—the Body Clutter that is in your head and heart. When we can fling this out, we can make room for the healing to begin, and along with it we can bring a smile back to your lovely face.

Please, open up your heart and put your arms around you! You deserve to be loved, and it all centers on the one love that cannot be taken from you—your love for yourself. If you don't do it, who will? Throughout this book we have given you simple, little changes to make in your life to help you with your attitudes as well as ways to be kind to yourself. Start taking those BabySteps to loving yourself. "Love" is a verb! Use every action in your power to show yourself that you are worth it! We know you can do this. We are cheering you on with each BabyStep that you take. We don't expect you to jump on this Body Clutter bandwagon with both feet. We have all crashed and burned with new books and ideas. We just want you to implement a few things in your daily and weekly routines. When those become established habits or, shall we say, lifestyle changes, then you can add other effective habits to your routines.

From the time we were little children, we have been told that if you can't do something right, don't do it at all. This kind of thinking is what got our home and body in the chaotic state that seems to overwhelm us. This is perfectionism!

We have been taught that perfect was the only way to be. This perfectionism has infiltrated every area of our lives: home, family, school, church, friendships, work, housework, yard work, leisure time, and our body.

As women, we were led to believe that we could have it all. We could bring home the bacon and fry it up in a pan. We could be the perfect wife, mother, and executive. But this didn't leave much room for being you, did it?

It wasn't as if we had someone standing over us with a whip expecting us to be good little wives and mothers. We were the ones holding ourselves up to standards that no one can live up to. Oh, we think we have seen women who seem to be everything to everyone, but do you ever see them smile when no one is looking? Our perfectionism is killing us one relationship at a time; that perfectionism makes us miserable—we don't even like ourselves.

In our perfectionism, we tell our husbands that their help is not good enough. If our ugly words do not deflate their loving gesture of folding towels, our action of refolding them will tell them loud and clear that their help is not good enough. Our children have to deal with this all the time, too.

You have said it time and again, "Go clean your room!" They proceed to clean, then you come in and take over! And with words that cut to the heart, "I might as well do it myself; you can never do anything right! Why bother asking you to do it?"

Eventually your perfectionism starts eating away at you. You keep juggling all the things that you think you have to do and then all of a sudden you can't keep all those plates spinning without some of them hitting the floor. Your perfectionism is the reason you have all those plates spinning in the first place. You volunteer for jobs that you don't think anyone else can do as well as you can. Your perfectionism won't allow you to say no! Before you know it, something begins to suffer. Most of the time it is your family that you neglect; the house gets messy and you can't tell it no, either. So your family is told they can't go to the park because you have to do the dishes or the laundry needs attention. All the while it is your poor family that really needs the attention but you have been giving it first to many other things.

Now here is the result of this neglect. You begin to feel guilty because your perfectionism is beating you up! You end up calling yourself lazy because you hear yourself utter all those unending excuses. Let's just call it what it really is—whining! No one loves a whiner! Not even you! The guilt gets worse and you start getting sick and putting on a few pounds. You have been living on a steady dose of adrenaline all because your perfectionism is eating away at you or eating away the pain of being imperfect.

So who suffers the most? Your husband? Your children?

I think it is you! All you want is to be the perfect housewife and mother and, at the same time, an experienced professional. The problem is that no one ever told you how to do this!

Then we take a look in the mirror and we don't see perfect. We proceed to condemn everything we see and we start sinking deeper into our need for perfection. Do you see the vicious cycle that pain, perfectionism, and procrastination has you in? You don't like what you see or how you feel, so you turn to your only comfort, the one thing that makes you feel better—food. At the same time you beat yourself up with all the negative things that have ever been said to you by you or anyone else. Then you hear those words, "I don't have time," which means I don't have time to do it right! Then we procrastinate and eventually say, "Why bother!"

In our perfectionism, we want what we want and we want it *now*! We search high and low for the ellusive magic pill, get-organized potion, or miraculous diet. We think if we just buy enough books, tapes, and plastic organizers that somehow it will all get better. The truth is that it is not the diet or get-organized books, motivational tapes, or plastic organizers that help us out of the CHAOS and Body Clutter—it is you! You have to want peace in order to make simple changes in your life and let the perfectionism go once and for all. Your attitude is the key that unlocks all the books, tapes, and tools.

Perfectionism is everywhere; see it for what it really is: a standard that is unattainable by anyone and a disease of unhappiness. I received a message about my cartoon character after I had lost around forty pounds. Here is what it said:

*Dear FlyLady . . .*

*It is time that you changed that obviously obese FlyLady picture to the NEW FlyLady picture! Seeing this chubby lady that couldn't fly if she wanted to . . . does not represent the new spirit of flyLady.net. Give her some muscles . . . make her pleasingly thinNER . . .*
*NOT SKINNY . . .*

*Just a very valid opinion and suggestion.*
*FLYing in Virginia*

I have gotten a lot of bad messages over the years, but I guess this one takes the cake. I realize that she was not trying to be mean, but this hurt my feelings more than any other message I have ever received. Perfectionism is in every area of our lives.

It is the attitude that thin is more pleasing than fat, that fat people are stupid, uncoordinated, and somehow can't FLY that has me so upset. This is a misconception that has been created by the advertising world and our perfectionism. My weight loss has not been because I want to look better; it is so I can live to do what God put me on this earth to do.

I am going to have to take every hurtful phrase and break it down so you can see the evil that is perfectionism.

" . . . *obviously obese FlyLady picture*": Our cartoon

character was drawn from pictures of me in 2001. Yes, I know that I was obese then and I am obese now. It is obvious to everyone who has ever seen me in person that I am not a little woman. Up until the last few months I had been the same size for many years. I didn't gain or lose. I was a steady size twenty-two. It was so easy to buy clothes. That *"obviously obese FlyLady"* picture has warmed the hearts of lots of people because of her comforting eyes and her warm smile. She is loving in a noncondescending way. You look at her and you can just picture her wrapping her arms around you and how safe that would make you feel. She has a gentle way of shaking her mommy finger and telling you to take care of yourself. You can see how much she loves you all. She wants you to have the peace that she has. That peace didn't come from being *"pleasingly thinNER."* It came from FLYing.

*"Seeing this chubby lady that couldn't fly if she wanted to . . . does not represent the new spirit of flyLady.net":* There is no new spirit at FlyLady.net or in me. There is the same loving character that made me who I am. It didn't matter if I was fat or skinny, tall or short, brown-eyed or blue, black or white, Christian or Muslim, American or Italian, a stay-at-home mom or an executive, a woman or a man—anyone can FLY! It doesn't take being thin for you to succeed. All it takes is wanting to get rid of the CHAOS that you have been living in and establishing some simple routines while releasing your perfectionism.

This chubby lady did FLY, and she is continuing to FLY as she helps all of you get your wings. At the same time, she can be the loving wife, mother, grandmother, business-woman, friend, and FLYLADY!

*"Give her some muscles . . . "*: She already has the most powerful muscle of all—a heart that has the ability to love everyone. My cartoon character will never change. The cartoonist once morphed her into a sleazy-looking character. I absolutely pitched a fit. At that point I bought the copyright from him and made him remove her from his website. When you see her, I want you to feel the love that she has to offer, not a smug attitude.

She is who you need her to be! She is lots of things to all different people. She is a drill sergeant when you need directions, she is a fairy Godmother when you start seeing your home come together, she is a loving mother when you need scolding, and she is your biggest cheerleader. She always has on her pearls, tennis shoes, and a smile. Her hair is fixed and with those eyes she tells you that you are loved not because of your size but who you are inside. She loves you unconditionally. She is FlyLady. It is because she first loved herself that she can love you!

I hope you see that this is more than being critical of just me; it is how so many people automatically think. In their perfectionism they can't and don't love themselves. The other night I went to sleep praying for you all. I want you to find the peace that I have. This peace came from the simple routines that we teach you and from FLYing! Finally Loving Yourself is the foundation for this world. Love your neighbor as yourself, but you can't love her till you truly love yourself.

Many of us have lived with criticism our whole lives because of our SHEness and our weight. We are not what we do or how we look. We are who we are because of our loving spirit that is in our hearts. Don't allow those perfectionists to steal the joy from your life. They are stuck in their own torment, and until they can learn to FLY they are only going to continue to give backhanded compliments to make themselves feel superior.

Release your perfectionism! We are our own worst enemy when perfectionism is our foundation and not love! My cartoon character will never change—it doesn't matter if I get to be a size two. She is the loving spirit that is inside me and all of us. Embrace that spirit and open up your wings and FLY!

I love you all!
*FlyLady*

## Body Clutter Mission

Open up your Body Clutter Control Journal and write down exactly what you are feeling right this minute. You can do this! You have been practicing letting go of your perfectionism.

This is not the end of this book. It is the beginning of your Body Clutter journey.

If you don't do it—who will?